From Harriet
with Love

From Harriet with Love

Kit and John Davis

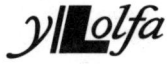

First impression: 2012

Cover design: Kit and John Davis and Y Lolfa

ISBN: 978 184771 419 0

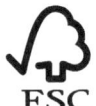

FSC

Published and printed in Wales
on paper from well maintained forests by
Y Lolfa Cyf., Talybont, Ceredigion SY24 5HE
website www.ylolfa.com
e-mail ylolfa@ylolfa.com
tel 01970 832 304
fax 832 782

To Harriet,
who was the inspiration for the formation of the
Charity which would enable families with disabled
children to take holidays together and all those, too
numerous to mention, who assisted in any way to
bring her wish to fruition.

Our special thanks must go to:

Dr Sandy Cavenagh for his interest and encouragement

Jenny Axon for typing the manuscript

Kevin Ayres for valuable technical advice

Those friends who have contributed their memories

Mats Lundalv of
Blissymbolics Communication International
for permitting the downloading and use of Blissymbols

Gwenda Jones of Ysgol Craig y Parc
for pointing us in the right direction

Contents

FOREWORD

by the Rt Rev. Dewi M Bridges MA

THE POET, C Day Lewis, wrote a poem entitled 'Walking Away for Sean', describing the parting of the ways which must take place in all families at some time or other. It ends with the lines:

> I have had worse partings, but none that so
> Gnaws in my mind still. Perhaps it is roughly
> Saying what God alone can perfectly show –
> How selfhood begins with walking away,
> And love is proved in the letting go.

More than 30 years ago some dear friends of mine, a priest and his doctor wife, were separated from the middle one of their three daughters when she got off the school bus outside the vicarage gate and ran into the path of an oncoming car. Helena was eight years old when her life ended prematurely. Her father, himself a poet, wrote in a book entitled *The Story of Helena* a poem to which he gave the title 'Love and Let Go, inspired by C Day Lewis': "And love is proved in the letting go."

The Swiss educationalist, J H Pestalozzi, devoted his life to the children of the very poor in the 18th century, coining the phrase, "Where love is, there God has his sanctuary." Another phrase that comes to mind is, "Love is never wasted." The story of Harriet is one of love, devotion and determination. *From Harriet with Love* is the story of the short life of just eleven years told by her parents Kit and John Davis, which includes contributions by a selection of others among the many who also loved and cared for her. I knew Harriet for but a fleeting moment when I visited her home in Llangynidr to administer the Sacrament of Confirmation not long before she died.

From Harriet with Love is a remarkable story which deserves to be told for the benefit of others as well as to provide a suitable tribute to Harriet's own life. If ever the truth of the saying "love is never wasted" needed justification, the story of Harriet proves it. It demonstrates how the story of a young person's life, "a life filled with love, laughter and happiness," can continue even after "love is proved in the letting go." Her wish, "I like to know that everyone has a holiday," is being achieved through the work of the Harriet Davis Seaside Holiday Trust for Disabled Children, which was set up in her memory. The needs of families with a disabled child for rest and recreation have been provided for in a remarkably creative and imaginative way for many years through the four houses owned by the Trust. The responses from those who have stayed in them provide ample evidence of the degree to which they are appreciated. "Where love is, there is God in his sanctuary." Harriet's life was both valuable and valued. May she rest in peace and rise in glory.

CHAPTER 1

Late Arrival

'Ah, dream too bright to last'
E A Poe (1809–1849) – 'To one in Paradise'

HAVING NEVER MADE much of our wedding anniversaries, or indeed the passing years, we felt that we should do something for our 50th, and so invited a number of friends to a lunch at Carringtons, our favourite restaurant in Tenby. The table plan was almost a roll-call of those who had played important parts in our daughter Harriet's life and the development of the Trust established in her name after her death. For instance: the two Angelas and their husbands who we met at the ante-natal clinic thirty years previously and whose sons, David, Gethyn, Gareth and Rhydian became Harriet's "best boys"; Roger, who tore apart two houses to adapt them for holiday houses for families with disabled children. Bishop Dewi Bridges and the Reverend Kelvin Richards, Harriet's spiritual advisors were there. Also in attendance, as so often in the past, were Harriet's medical team: Alva, Jan, Rose and Doctor Sandy. They and the others present, play an important part in this story together with the numerous other good people who helped along the way. During the meal, Sandy Cavenagh who had written a book about his experiences as the Medical Officer with the 3rd Para during the Suez crisis urged us, not for the first time, to write 'the book' and gave us a deadline for the first chapter.

In 1980 we were living near Brecon where we had been

working for some seven years. Brecon is a small market town, six thousand people lived there at that time. It was a widely held belief that there were more sheep than people in the county of Powys, which is an amalgamation of the old counties of Brecknockshire, Radnorshire and Montgomeryshire. To travel from one end of Powys to the other, John said, was equivalent to driving from the Severn Bridge to London. Very beautiful too, with the Beacons Mountains about the town, although harsh in places with the Army training and firing ranges on the Eppynt. The sparse population was scattered and village communities tight-knit. Has it changed much? Probably not. Brecon town has grown quite considerably in the last thirty years but the character of this part of Wales, in essence, remains unchanged.

It all began when Kit was completing her thesis for a Master's Degree in Education at Cardiff University. John was working as a Community Development Officer for Powys Education Authority in the south of the county. Kit was part of the peripatetic remedial team attached to the schools Psychology Service. She continues the story in her own words.

Part of my duties was to visit some six primary schools to give extra tuition to children who were falling below a certain level in their reading and mathematical skills. John's job involved him in organizing Adult Education and Adult Literacy classes. He also supervised the network of Youth and Community Centres in the area and, amongst other things, advised sports clubs and community groups on the sources of grants for village halls and sport facilities. Between us we knew and were known by many people in the town and county.

My thesis was based on a statistical analysis of data gathered from a piece of research that I had formulated and carried out into the nature and possible causes of failure in young children to learn mathematics. I had finished the work and was preparing to go down to the university for a viva examination of my findings by a visiting lecturer from London University. The day before this final hurdle I visited our GP's surgery where I had been on several previous visits with a general feeling of malaise. Probably overwork, a kidney infection, anxiety about my thesis were the general conclusions – except on this occasion. Perhaps I have another ovarian cyst? I ventured to the doctor. Twenty years previously I had been misdiagnosed as having an ectopic pregnancy. However the operation revealed a normal pregnancy and a large ovarian cyst. As a consequence of the subsequent removal of the offending cyst I suffered a miscarriage in very early pregnancy.

This time there was no cyst and I will never forget the conversation with Dr Arwyn Davies. After examining me he leant against the wall to support his sagging knees, "What would you say," he asked, "if I told you, you are pregnant?"

"It's late, I'm tired. I have to go for my viva tomorrow and I'm not in the mood for foolish jokes," was my reply.

"I mean it. I mean it," he insisted. "Where's John?"

John was still in the office and when summoned was equally dumbfounded. We had been married for twenty years. I was forty-two and definitely almost at the end of an early menopause.

"Have you been drinking?" was my mother's response when John broke the news to her. Grossly unfair, as we were virtually a teetotal household. I survived the viva, probably because I was still in a state of disbelief.

We went for a scan and spread the news. Being nearly seven months pregnant and living in a small cottage on the Old Drovers' Road underneath the Storey Arms in the Brecon Beacons was not going to be easy. We had already been looking for a house that my mother could share with us, and it became even more important to find somewhere suitable. We have all heard or read stories of women who go unsuspectingly to hospital with a stomach ache (or something similar) and come home with a baby. I had always found this incredible. I believe it now. I was so very nearly one of that number.

When Harriet was born in October 1980 everyone commented on how beautiful she was. I thought that she looked like a small skinned rabbit, but as I had never been very interested in babies, I didn't voice my opinion. She was, however, quite small and fitted neatly into dolly's clothes donated by the daughter of Eddy Collier, one of John's colleagues. We went home from hospital and the journey began.

Visitors came to wonder and admire. Amongst the first was Dr Arwyn, standing in the doorway and smiling with relief and pleasure. We moved to a house in Llangynidr on a bitterly cold day when Harriet was a month old. A bitterly cold day, two cats, baby, me, exhausted and bewildered by the unexpected turn in my life and with a raging tooth abscess. The removal men asked "Where shall we put this packing case?" I begged them to just put my bed up and dragged myself there with the cats for mutual comfort, leaving my mother and John to look after everything else.

Mother produced the family christening robe. John asked Richard Evans, the Youth Chaplain and Vicar of St David's, Llanddew, if he would officiate at a christening service in his church. My cousin Susan, with whom my sister and I had grown up, came up from Cornwall with her husband, Kenny Rogers, Vicar of St George's Church in Truro, who assisted at the service. St David's, in the village of Llanddew, near Brecon, is a small church of great antiquity. Ogwen Thomas, County Music Advisor, and one of John's colleagues played the organ. The church was full with the rest of our family and friends who came from near and far. The singing was enthusiastic and uplifting. The Castle of Brecon Hotel provided tea and cake for everyone after the service. Brecon itself seemed to be 'en-fete'.

I freely acknowledge the debt that I owe to my mother and John for the fact that during the next few weeks I was helped to adjust to all the changes in my life. Harriet firmly established herself in my heart. Everybody was right, she was beautiful and good and growing at the rate of an inch a month. I made plans to return to work. Mrs Ella Price (Nana) from the village, agreed to come in to look after Harriet. Ella was assured, experienced and calm. Mother could return home to sell her house. It was sorted and under control.

CHAPTER 2

Troubled Times

'Alas regardless of their doom
The little victims play
No sense have they of ills to come,
Nor care beyond today!'
Thomas Gray – 'Ode on a
Distant Aspect of Eton College' (1747)

THERE IS A splendid irony in that my early fears about handling a baby, coping with the hitherto unknown routines of feeding and bathing, seemed unfounded. My return to the classroom went smoothly and, with Nana Price's expertise, all was well. Like Thomas Gray's little victims I had no sense of the ills to come.

The outset of H's illness was insidious. After a minor viral infection, quite common in infancy, Harriet began to lose ground. Feeding became difficult; her ability to sit up started to diminish. She developed a squint which then disappeared as suddenly as it had happened. I took her each week to the health clinic and when she began to lose weight with increasing rapidity, the feeling of sick heaviness in my stomach became panic and dread. The ensuing months passed in a blur. Every time I shake the kaleidoscope of memory a different moment is highlighted. We went to Dr Sandy Cavenagh, a fellow member of Brecon Lions' Club with John, who set us on the road of discovery. Going to Neville Hall Hospital in Abergavenny to see the Paediatric Consultant, the marvellous Dr Tony Griffiths, I remember him saying, "I know which book I want to look in but I am not sure which chapter. Bring Harriet onto the children's ward."

Within a week he had made a firm diagnosis. By the end of March 1982 we had been to Great Ormond Street Children's Hospital at Dr Griffiths' insistence that we seek a second opinion. He had only once before seen a child with Harriet's condition and didn't want us to have doubts about his diagnosis.

Mike Chamberlain, a colleague of John's, drove us to London. The diagnosis of Leigh's Encephalmyelopathy was confirmed. A very rare degenerative brain condition, in which, we learnt from the doctors, the brain stem would gradually die as the myelin sheaths around the nerve cells were destroyed by Harriet's own metabolism. The prognosis was bleak. A few months of progressive loss of physical abilities before inevitable death. No treatment. No cure.

During our stay at Great Ormond Street we were visited by a man who was unknown to us then, but who has since played a fundamental part in Harriet's story. At that time my sister was working as a micro-biologist at the Loseley Estate near Guildford in Surrey. There she had set up the laboratory as part of the growth of the Loseley ice-cream and yoghurt products. Loseley is an historic estate, mentioned in the Domesday Book and held by the More-Molyneux family since 1508 when it was bought by Sir Christopher More. In 1946 when James More-Molyneux inherited the estate it was in his words "dilapidated and struggling". In his book *The Loseley Challenge* James tells the story of his stewardship of the estate and describes the hard work of recovery and the development of its success.

My sister, Joan, told James about Harriet's illness and prognosis. She felt that she should resign from her position at Loseley in order to be available to help us care for Harriet whenever needed. All we knew of this was that James arrived at Great Ormond Street and asked us what did we need? Should he leave his car for us to use? Did we need any money?

In the years that followed, James and his wife Sue, came to Llangynidr to offer spiritual and practical help. The former we needed then, more than the latter.

We came to know James as a shy, unassuming man, a complex character, who was successful in business ventures which were underpinned with his steadfast and deep Christian faith. On a memorable visit to Guildford we took Harriet to Loseley and, with James, went into their Chapel where he prayed for her and for us. But all of that, and the part that James and Sue played during the formation of the Holiday Trust, lay in the future.

We stayed in Great Ormond Street for a week, maybe longer. During this time we were asked if Harriet could be the subject of a seminar with consultants, doctors and others, because her condition was so rare. Despite her fragile state we agreed, but were anxious about the additional stress on her already weakened body. Harriet's ability to swallow was failing rapidly and she was quickly becoming increasingly frail. We were afraid that she would die so far from home. We decided to return to Wales and Neville Hall Hospital. Exhausted and emotionally drained as we both were, our reception on arrival at the children's ward was wonderful. A mother and baby room was ready and waiting. "Welcome Home," I don't remember who said those words but that was how it felt. We were surrounded by capable and loving support. Rose Hopkins, who had been the very first to greet us on our initial visit to the ward, was there. Under her encouraging, calm instruction I learnt to pass a nasogastric tube so that Harriet could receive some nutrition and fluid. We returned home to await the inevitable.

We have never questioned "Why us? Why our child?" We were not the first parents to be faced with losing an only child. It is not our intention to write in detail about neither the progress of Harriet's illness nor the minutiae of coping with her frailty, frequent chest infections and poor body temperature control. There are so many medical emergencies and problems that are part and parcel of Leigh's disease. Countless parents experience similar with other disabilities and learn to cope, as we did, to a lesser or greater extent. Very early on, Dr Cavenagh asked me how what we were experiencing fitted in or affected my philosophy of life. At that time, I didn't have an answer, except rather baldly to say "I don't have a philosophy". Thirty years on, I realise that Harriet's life and death have profoundly altered my approach to, and expectations from, my own life.

Harriet's life span of almost twelve years far exceeded predictions. Throughout that time we received tremendous support from the staff at Neville Hall. It is a tribute to everyone involved in Harriet's care that we continue to keep in touch. We still have news of Sister Rosemary, Sister Joan and Sister Anna – now all retired from the children's ward. Rose Hopkins, who visited Harriet every week, continues to be an important part of our life. Harriet and I were frequent visitors to the children's ward and it became a place where she felt comfortable and easy because everyone was so kind to her.

Harriet's paediatric physiotherapist, Jan Boreham, and the night nurse, Alva Corbett, became a part of our family as did Maureen Probert the health visitor. Marion Lewis, who had taken the antenatal classes, came regularly in the latter years to give H acupuncture which seemed to give some relief from pain. When Harriet caught the measles, probably because she had had only the first part of the triple vaccine before the onset of the Leigh's disease, everyone rallied round. My sister, Joan, came to stay during this time. I was scheduled to have an operation on my wrist because of a painful carpel tunnel condition. I went to Brecon Hospital where Dr Dimyian, assisted by Uncle Sandy (Dr Cavenagh), performed the operation under a local anaesthetic. I was invited to 'have a look' as they worked – but my kept my eyes firmly fixed anywhere but at the exposed workings of my wrist. I was able to return home later that same day. I knew that I would be unable to use my hand for at least two weeks. During the course of Harriet's illness her temperature rose dramatically. My sister needed to sleep. I had the use of only one hand. It was before Alva had been engaged to help. In despair I phoned Maureen Probert who lived on the farm at the very end of a two-mile narrow road up into the Cwm Crawnon Valley. It was, I remember, a cold frosty night. She rolled out of bed, telling her half-awake husband, "I'm going down to Harriet's." We spent the rest of the night tending to the patient and were relieved when just after dawn her temperature dropped to a more manageable level.

At this point Harriet shared our bedroom. My sister, John and I took it in turns to sleep in the spare room, or in my mother's bed during the day. I vividly remember John asking rather plaintively one morning, "Which bed is free now? Can I have a sleep?" During these early months and years my mother sold her house and moved in with us permanently and a small extension was built giving her a sitting room, bedroom and shower room. Sadly Nana Price died within a very short while of our return from Great Ormond Street, giving us another loss to grieve over.

I received my Master's degree from Cardiff University but by now my plans to continue and develop the research further to form the basis of a doctorate seemed of no importance and to belong to another life, certainly not mine. I was given extended leave of absence from work and, despite everything, we settled into something close to a routine.

CHAPTER 3

What do you do all day?

'Monday's child is fair of face,
Tuesday's child is full of grace,
Wednesday's child is full of woe...'
A E Bray – *Traditions of Devonshire* (1838)

THERE ARE A great many metabolic diseases, some are common and treatments have been developed over the years; Diabetes is but one example. Other inborn errors of metabolism such as Leigh's Encephalomyelopathy are very rare and often referred to as orphan diseases. This is because the odds against two people carrying the same recessive gene meeting and marrying are very long. The chances of any child of this union developing the defective gene as a full-blown disease are usually one in four. Even more rarely is there medical research into any one specific orphan disease. No cure, no treatment and a bleak prognosis. Harriet was born on Wednesday, 29th October 1980. It seemed to us that she was indeed full of woe. We mourned for the child that might have been as we struggled to establish some routine in our lives.

Six months had passed since the initial diagnosis of Leigh's disease. Defying the prognosis of two months of rapid decline ending in death, Harriet clung on to life, frail but, unbelievably, still alive.

I came to the decision that, in order to retain my own sanity, the crying must stop. Harriet's life, however long or short, should not be full of woe. If nothing else there would be music, stories, a bright and cheerful house with much to look at and the company of friends to share and laugh with.

Gradually a team of helpers began to form. Probably the first was the paediatric physiotherapist, Jan Boreham. As with most aspects of H's life it was a small and not particularly ambitious start and to do what was necessary to keep her comfortable was the remit: postural drainage to help keep her lungs clear from infection, simple passive exercises to keep her more comfortable and aid her ability to sit. Jan came twice a week for routine sessions and at many other times, official and unofficial, when Harriet was poorly with yet another chest infection. Sunday or Christmas Day, Jan never seemed to mind.

Jan and her family lived close by in Llangynidr and her husband, Ivan, taught at the secondary school in Crickhowell. Gradually their family became part of the warp and weft of our lives. Harriet obviously enjoyed her physio sessions and showed great determination and courage. Pursuing my decision to act as if Harriet would have a normal life span and experience as much as possible, we listened to nursery rhymes, sang songs to her, read stories and looked at books together.

We walked for miles along the village lanes with a carriage-sprung old pram borrowed, I believe, from the children's ward at Neville Hall Hospital. Propped up in this roomy, smooth-running chariot, Harriet had a good view of everything around her. Llangynidr was once described as being on the road from nowhere to nowhere. It certainly lacks a bus service but is indisputably in a very beautiful part of mid Wales. The village is surrounded by farmland and hills, with wonderful views across the valley to the Sugar Loaf Mountain. The River Usk marks the lower village boundary and the Brecon and Monmouth canal runs through the middle of the village. On our walks there was always plenty of wildlife to see, as well as horses and sheep in the fields. We became a familiar sight when the weather was fine and people would stop and chat or smile and say hello to us as we explored the paths around the village. Ted and Albert Price, two veterans of the locality (and of the 'local') would jokingly beg a lift in the chariot as they ambled homewards after a pint or two in the Coach and Horses Inn. The village shop, the Post Office, the canal path, top chapel, bottom chapel and church, all were markers along our way.

Incredibly small improvements in Harriet became noticeable. I remember the day that she moved her arms and hands in response to specific instructions, demonstrating some mobility skill but also verbal understanding and body image; for example we now knew that Harriet understood where her knees were and could place her hands on them. She became able to lift her head a little and turn it to look left and right without visual clues. Her targeting skills with her hands improved. These small, but significant, abilities showed quite unequivocally that, although her mobility was grossly impaired, intellectually a brain was busy working. I needed to discover the best ways to unlock this intelligence. I felt rather like the hapless mariner in A A Milne's poem, 'The Old Sailor':

> There was once an old sailor my Grandfather knew
> Who had so many things which he wanted to do
> That whenever he thought it was time to begin
> He couldn't because of the state he was in.

Shipwrecked on a remote island the old man could not decide what to do first; make a hat or some trousers, or a hook to catch fish, look for water, make a hut and so on.

> So in the end he did nothing at all
> But basked on the shingle wrapped up in a shawl...

until he was rescued. I had no such luxury of time, as no-one was going to come and rescue me. I had to keep on juggling all the many tasks if we were to make any progress.

John Prout came into our lives when Harriet outgrew her chariot and we also wanted something more manageable to take on trips to town and elsewhere. John runs a business, D C S Joncare (based near Oxford), supplying equipment for children with special needs. We first met in Cardiff where he had come to demonstrate a brand new 'buggy' manufactured by a Swedish company. This was a whole new concept in the care of a child with special needs. Something that was easy to transport, looking more like a 'normal' buggy, yet suitable for children like H. The Swedish name 'Sulky', at first seemed inauspicious, with its overtones of sullen moroseness. On reflection I realised that the *Oxford Reference Dictionary* also gives its meaning as 'a light two-wheeled horse-drawn vehicle for one – especially used in trotting races'. An apt name then after all, even if the horse (me) lacked the fine lines and speed of a trotting pony. The snag with the 'Sulky' was that it had not yet been approved for use by the health authorities and they were unwilling to fund its purchase. A certificate, we learned, would take at least a year to be granted. We felt that this was the buggy for H and, after much haggling, it was agreed that if we signed an indemnity absolving the authorities from any blame if an accident occurred, they would sanction the purchase. We duly did this, emerging victorious from our first encounter with the bureaucracy of disability. The first, sadly, of many such encounters.

Jumping to the future, in 1994 we were coming out of the first Trust holiday house, "Harriet's House" at the harbour in Tenby. It must have been during the autumn and we were visiting from Brecon to see how things were going – certainly no family was staying there on that day. As we came through the front door we saw three people reading the plaque fixed to the wall by the door:

Harriet's House
The Harriet Davis Seaside Holiday Trust for Disabled Children

We invited them in to look at what we had done. Whilst there, and in the course of conversation, we realised that we had met the man of the group somewhere before. It was none other than John Prout, last seen in 1983! He was on holiday, visiting relatives still living in the nearby village of Stepaside where John had been raised. Our association has not faltered since then and we have purchased much of our special seating equipment from his company. The chapel his sister attends in Stepaside has supported the cause with donations, and we now find ourselves living very close to Stepaside village. It is often said that the world of disability is very small. Upon coincidental events like these such truisms are founded.

CHAPTER 4

On the Move: of Wheelchairs and Moulds

'Are you sitting comfortably?'
Listen With Mother, BBC Radio Programme

A GOOD SITTING position is fundamental to many learning situations. Of equal importance is its role in the physical wellbeing and skeletal development of the growing child who is unable to walk or support any part of his or her body unaided: enter the Patient Support Unit at Rookwood Hospital in Cardiff. Dr Chris Barr ran this small unit. He and his team made specialised seating moulds for patients with complex physical disabilities and needs. Thirty years ago this unit was at the van of research and design. Harriet must have been one of his earliest and youngest referrals. How lucky we were to be part of this development. We would travel down to Cardiff and spend a day in the workshop while measurements were taken and positioning considered at length. It was far from a clinical, sterile environment but again we felt we were both part of an exciting new development and reassured by Chris's skill and warm personality. A little dust in the atmosphere was of no importance.

H's first seating moulds were made of interlocking pieces – several hundred, probably – fitted together to give her the right support. Chris and his team would, on occasion, come to our home to make final adjustments. This could take several hours. Harriet would lie, propped on the settee, and under her eagle eye the floor became a sea of meccano-like pieces while the experts worked to achieve the best possible fit. Mr Pod, Chris's part-Husky part-German shepherd dog, would sit patiently or lie outside in the garden until Harriet was sitting in the finished mould. A foam liner, which we further covered with a natural lamb's fleece, made the mould more comforting. It was then fitted into a standard child-sized wheelchair and secured with clips. Later, moulds entirely of foam rubber were developed by Chris and great improvements made to head rests. Young, inventive and caring, Dr Barr and his team gave Harriet the chance to see the world around her from a more normal perspective. It opened up the opportunity for her to learn and develop such skills as she had for as long or short a time as she might have. We wish we could record that Chris continued his sterling work at Rookwood but, at some point, he took an inviting offer to develop his work further in North America. Whilst there, and still a young man, he died suddenly of a hitherto undetected heart defect. We remember him with great affection and gratitude.

During the early 1980s the choice of wheelchairs into which special seating moulds could be fitted was limited. Even more limited in vision was official understanding of the needs of the disabled in general and of growing children in particular. Funding of equipment sadly continues to be a contentious issue and delays in supplying properly fitting seating to keep pace with physical growth causes parents and carers as much worry and frustration today as we experienced, thirty years ago.

Early in 1986, when H was five years old we felt that she had progressed sufficiently to be given the chance to try an electric wheelchair. This gave rise to a real chicken and egg situation. In order to qualify for a NHS-funded chair, she had first demonstrate that she had the ability to drive and stop when asked. A bit like having to pass your road test to drive a car before being allowed to take driving lessons. We pointed out that it was an impossible demand unless H was first given a battery operated chair which, not only had a special seating mould fitted for her, but which also had controls adapted to suit her. It was an impasse – a vicious circle of the first order. In desperation we began to research into the type and availability of a chair that we might buy privately. It was like entering unknown territory without map or compass and complicated by the fact we had only a hazy idea of the destination: a battery-operated chair that Harriet could both sit in and drive. Was it a real possibility, or merely an unrealistic dream? All this happened before the explosion of information provided by the internet which everyone now takes almost for granted. It was more difficult then for the non-professional to research and access specialist information.

All the illustrations we looked at seemed to show children with far better physical ability than Harriet. John found an emerging company, based in Cambridge, which had developed a wheelchair on which the height and tilt of the seat could be altered. This innovative chair was called the Turbo. A trip to Cambridge was mooted. It might as well have been a trip to the moon. It was not the actual mileage that was daunting, but the amount of baggage needed – suction machine and portable oxygen cylinder, medicines, feed, clothing. We would need nearly as much for one night away from home, as for a week. We stayed overnight near Cambridge with some friends from our time teaching in Haverhill, Suffolk during the late 1960s. The landscape of East Anglia is greatly different from Wales. No mountains but acres of huge crop fields under vast skyscapes. Later, in her diary, Harriet remembered the "happy yellow fields" of rapeseed in full vivid chrome-yellow coloured flower.

After seeing the Turbo wheelchair we felt that we had found the answer to our problems. Once back home we reported to Jan, Harriet's physiotherapist, that we believed the chair could be suitable. Harriet's seating mould could be fitted to it and the controls modified sufficiently so that she could learn to drive.

All we had to do to enable Harriet to be the proud owner of a bright red customised Turbo wheelchair was to find the several thousand pounds purchase price. During the third week of June 1986, Jan and her husband asked us if we could walk along to the Coach and Horses Inn, about half a mile away from our house, close by the canal. "Sunday morning," she said, "a few friends are going to have a fun run in aid of research into heart disease in children. It would be lovely if Harriet could come and start them off." So, on a Sunday morning, we set off for the pub. Rose came with us. As we rounded the bend in the road just before the pub, we were amazed to see a huge crowd of people, all wearing running numbers pinned to their chests, waiting for us. Harriet was presented with the number 1 to fix on the front of her wheelchair tray.

This fun run had been an extraordinarily well-kept secret from us. The money raised was not only for research, as we had been told, but mainly to go towards Harriet's new wheels. Over 700 runners took part and the circular route around the village, whilst not lengthy at about three and a half miles, had a lot of uphill ground to be covered. The runners ranged from a baby in a pram, toddlers accompanied by their parents, to serious runners. One pensioner of some 80 years completed the circuit, as did the doughty veterans Ted and Albert Price and Alf Puncher. These three were already known to Harriet as we met them along the back lanes on our walks. As well as villagers people came from all around: Crickhowell, Abergavenny and Brecon were well represented. Harriet's friends, Gethyn and David, were there with their parents and granny, as well as many other friends. At the end of the day enough money had been raised for us to buy the Turbo wheelchair.

The whole event had been organized for 26 June at 11.30 a.m. by Jan's husband, Ivan, together with three other locals: John Gregory, Byron Llewellyn and Sean James. There was live music from a jazz group and a barbeque where young Royal Navy personnel from HMS Collingswood on a course nearby were the cooks. Police Inspector Ralph Reece supervised the temporary road closure. Legend has it that when John regretted that the pub was closed (no all-day opening in the 1980s) the senior policeman promptly gave an early doors order. Whether or not this was true Kit is unable to confirm, as Harriet and mother were on the way back home by then. What a day. Seven hundred runners, plus nearly as many supporters, music, laughter, and food. Even the time of the morning service in church was brought forward so that the congregation could attend or run. We will not forget such kindness or the memory of shock and pleasure when the surprise was sprung as we came around that bend in the road.

In her daybook for 1986, Harriet recorded her thoughts about many things including where she had been and how she was feeling. The entry for 5 July has a picture of the Turbo, "I want new chair." When asked, "What will you do when you have it?" her reply was that she would be "Happy, see my friends." On 19 July, getting impatient: "When chair come?" "My new chair!" On Wednesday, 20 August, her question is "When from shop comes my chair?" At last on Saturday, 8 November, "The new chair I have."

Later in December, difficulties in getting the controls were recorded but Turbo was undoubtedly a huge success. John had a special number plate made to fix on the back: H.D.1. Not that there was much danger of mistaken identity with such a striking chariot.

Gradually Harriet learnt to manage the adapted controls. Backward circles down the slope of the cul-de-sac of our road, or ever-increasing circles on the bumpy recreation field – all done at maximum speed – gave her great satisfaction and increased heart rates in those of us anxiously watching her progress. A basket fixed atop the battery housing at the back of the chair, held the suction machine and away we went. The village lanes, already explored in our pram pushing days became her familiar walks. The horses came to the gateway to greet her. One year, at the annual village gala day, Harriet and Jennifer from next door, entered the fancy dress parade as 'Meals on Wheels'. With a sunshade fixed to the back of her seat, the wheels decorated with menus, a cup and saucer secured on her tray Harriet was accompanied by 'nippy' waitress Jennifer. Resplendent in lace pinny and cap, Jennifer's wheels were provided by the roller skates strapped to her feet. They won a well deserved prize, reflecting appreciation not only of the originality and aptness of the idea, but of the fact that they managed not to run anyone down or bruise any shins, other than Jennifer's, during the afternoon.

Turbo opened up more and more opportunities for Harriet. Today, probably, the words 'equal' and 'access' would feature somewhere. The terminology is immaterial. The new wheelchair allowed Harriet to take a more active part in the life of our community as much as she was able, and so her life experience was further enriched.

A portable ramp into the church made by Major Mike Dyer and covered, of course, with red carpet, was Harriet's next test of driving skill. The slope down from the porch into the body of the church was quite steep, but she accomplished it with great élan and a satisfying thump as she came off the end of the ramp. She loved to 'sing' along, and the congregation never seemed to mind that or the noise of the suction machine when it was needed. In the winter, when she was well enough to go out (or if the weather was too cold to be outside), we would visit one of the large supermarkets with wide aisles to practise circuit driving at quiet times. Staff and customers on these occasions appeared to find us quite unremarkable and paid us scant attention.

CHAPTER 5

Can you hear me?

'I long to talk'
John Donne (1572–1631) – 'Loves Deity'
from *Songs and Sonnets*

FOR A NUMBER of years we had a poster fixed to a wall in our living room. It was one issued by the organization now known as SCOPE which is concerned with people who have cerebral palsy. The picture showed a young girl in a wheelchair sitting in front of a computer. On the screen were the words: "Just because I couldn't talk they thought I had nothing to say." The challenge for us was to find a way to allow Harriet to 'speak'. In spite of all her motor disabilities, we felt sure that her intellect and capacity to learn was not yet damaged by the disease. One of the cruellest things about Leigh's disease is the random nature of its progress. It can affect any part of the body and progress in a series of decline and plateau. The plateau that Harriet was living on was to last for several years and she became neither blind nor deaf, or lost her mental faculties. Kit refused to believe that Harriet was incapable of learning to communicate.

Language development is a complex process and a necessary part of communication skills. Kit thought that the ability to make a choice would be a starting point. First, a choice between two things – standing in front of her and showing her two toys for example: "Which toy would you like? The white rabbit or baby Ted?"

Each toy was shown to her in turn and then held far enough apart to make it clear which one she looked at first. That one was given to her to touch or put into her arms. We progressed to three items placed on the table in front of her. Jan and the occupational therapist made an arm splint so that Harriet could begin to indicate choice by first pointing. Now her bow of choice had two strings to it – eye pointing and fist pointing.

The Special Education Media Resource Centre, based at Bristol, gave us great help. This resource centre for special education needs helped to find very touch-sensitive switches and widen our knowledge of what was available. We borrowed toys from their lending 'library'. These would all move by means of an attached and very sensitive switch. The lightest touch would start the toy into motion: a dog that turned somersaults, a hopping rabbit and a penguin slide (lent by a generous young friend) were favourites. A large yellow crane proved the most attractive. A small switch panel operated the arm – up, down, right, left. It was a big success and many happy times were spent picking up small loads onto the platform and placing them in trucks before sending them to another destination.

Soon we were holding what was in effect an at-home Mother and toddler group. Rhys, Jennifer, Gareth and Rhydian would come to join in the fun and take turns with the toys. The crane spent longer with us than anywhere else. At the same time we listened to music and read stories, painted (i.e. our hands became smothered in poster paint – some of which eventually got transferred to a sheet of sugar paper).

At some point Jan, the physiotherapist, felt that leg splints, boots and a standing frame would be possible and help Harriet's physical development. Every day, when well enough, some time could be spent in an upright position and many activities undertaken. Cake making was a favourite – most of the hard work was done by Kit in mixing the ingredients, but Harriet always enjoyed holding the wooden spoon and aiming it into the bowl. Kit always felt that the 'dribble' that went into the mixture added a little *je ne sais quoi* to the taste when cooked!

Nobody ever complained of ill effects afterwards – probably a high oven temperature took care of that.

We went to the hydrotherapy pool at Penmaes Special School in Brecon. It was not something that we were able to do for long, as it seemed to tire Harriet too much and her difficulties in swallowing made it a rather anxious time for everyone. Eventually Kit decided that the benefits for Harriet were not sufficiently great to continue. However, we did meet and make a new friend at the pool. Jo Blackburn was the organizer of the pre-school playgroups and became a firm friend, together with her family of four children. Harriet was learning to socialise with her own age group and, even if she couldn't speak, she was learning to communicate using those abilities that she had.

A young doctor in training once asked Kit "But what do you do all day?" Kit told him some of the activities that filled each day – physiotherapy, learning to communicate, going out for walks, indeed everything we did was merely an adaptation of what every pre-school child does (or should do).

We had reached the point where Kit felt that a more structured approach to communication and reading skills could be tackled.

It would have been about this time that 'Care in the Community' became a government philosophy. Kit's mother was showing signs of the cancer that was to end her life and for some weeks needed nursing at home as her ability to walk began to decline. At this point cancer had not been diagnosed but some problem with the vertebrae was suspected. For several weeks we managed to look after both mother and Harriet. John discovered, almost by accident in a casual conversation that there were two home-care assistants employed by Brecon Social Services for whom no work had been found. Even after all these years we find it hard to be complimentary about the support that we received from the Social Services and some tiers of the different branches of local and health authorities and government departments.

What saddens us is that many of the battles for support that we fought and won are still being fought by individual families today. The first of Harriet's home-carers came to help us on a daily basis. There were no barriers raised to Harriet being educated at home. Indeed, we were told that because of her physical condition formal tuition would be a waste of time. We could almost hear the sigh of relief from the Education Office – from then on Kit neither asked for, nor was offered, any real help from those in the authority. The Education Committee was, however, kind in granting Kit an extended leave of absence which eventually was regularised to enable her to claim a part pension in 1988.

We went to see the eye specialist at Neville Hall to see if Harriet needed glasses to help her read, as Kit and her sister were both short-sighted, as their father had been. We were astounded to be told that Harriet was blind. Kit wept all the way home. We just could not believe what we had been told. Everyone who knew Harriet was equally disbelieving. "Rubbish" we said. If H was blind, how could she look and choose, work the crane switch when asked to choose the correct one to make its arm move to right and left? We asked numerous such questions and decided that we could not accept the verdict. From all our observations we were positive that H could see. Chanting that well-known mantra, 'Mother knows best' we ignored the professionals and carried on as before. If we had not done so, this story would have been very different. Perhaps the creation of the Holiday Trust would never have come about.

But how to find the best way to unlock Harriet's skills? What was the key to help her progress? Reading skills normally develop quite slowly and, although Kit had experience of teaching children with the ability to speak, how to read, and how to teach those who found it difficult to learn the skills involved, she had never taught a child who was physically unable to speak. Harriet was at the age when she would normally have started full-time education – but she had a disease, which could have delayed her intellectual development – we had no real idea of how far she would be able to progress or how long a time she had ahead. The effects of Leigh's disease can be very varied: one child might be blind, another deaf, one would be able to swallow, another not, and so on. Once again we decided to go ahead as if the situation would remain either static or improve, and as if Harriet would live a normal life span. Self-deluding such an approach might be, but better that than sitting and doing nothing.

After a little research the name Bliss came to the surface. Charles Bliss was a refugee from Nazi anti-Semitic persecution during the Second World War. During the time he spent living in Shanghai, he became familiar with Chinese Ideograms. After the war in 1949, when he was fifty-three years of age, Bliss wanted to create an easy to learn universal written language to allow communication between people speaking different native languages. The system he envisaged would both augment a person's native language and be clear and unambiguous in meaning. In 1949, then, Bliss published his theory and system of 'World Writing' explaining what the exact layout and structure of this system should be.

Bliss was disappointed that his system did not become universally popular. It did however find increasing favour as a method of alternative communication and language for those who, for one reason or another, were physically unable to speak. Indeed, initially, he sued some centres teaching his system to cerebral palsy sufferers and accepted an out-of-court settlement. In 1971 Bliss symbols were used with children for the first time. This was at the Ontario Crippled Children's Centre in Toronto, Canada. Bliss had by now obviously accepted the inevitable use of his system with non-speaking children and worked with a draughtsman, Jim Grice, and Margaret Beesley from the Centre, to ensure that the pictures would be consistent in their presentation to children. The Crippled Children's Centre is now known as the Bloorview Kids Rehab.

In 1975 a new organization named Bliss Symbolics Communication Foundation was set up and continues, with various changes of name, as Blissymbolics Communication International. It is strange to think that when Charles Bliss died in 1985 at the age of eighty-eight, Harriet was five years old and about to benefit from his legacy.

Kit borrowed weighty volumes about the Bliss system via the inter-library loan service, delivered almost to the door by that wonderful mobile library scheme which still operates in very rural areas. The books were scholastic in approach and offered almost too much information. We needed face-to-face advice from teachers already using the system. We liked the views that we read: that speech and language therapists and users felt that children who learn to communicate with Blissymbolics find it easier to learn to read and write traditional script and spelling in their own language than those who do not. Kit felt that it would offer Harriet a means of developing her language, learning new words, new concepts and grammar while her reading skills could develop at a slower rate. There are those experts who believe that true ideographic writing systems with the same capacities as natural language do not exist. We didn't have time to worry about the semantics of the theory. Once again, we had reached a blind corner and did not know fully what lay ahead. Success, failure or something in between.

CHAPTER 6

Word Search

'Words are but the signs of ideas'
Samuel Johnson – *Dictionary of the English language* (1753)

THOSE WORDS OF Samuel Johnson are a self-evident truth and particularly apposite for us as we came to grips with the world of Blissymbols.

"What I need," said Kit, "is some expert help," and sent John off to find it. John's research skills were getting plenty of practice and were being honed to a highly polished finish. Locked away from Harriet in his office, with a phone in one hand and a cigarette in the other, he could somehow find the answers to all demands for information. Complete strangers on the receiving end of his enquiries quickly became firm friends and freely gave advice and help.

He made contact with Craig-y-Parc School near Cardiff, a residential and day school for about 40 children with severe learning difficulties where Bliss symbols were used. The staff there were so helpful and kind. After a day's visit with Harriet, we came away with a firmer idea of where to start, a chart of the most useful symbols to teach and an assurance that we were welcome to go back at any time if we needed more help.

Kit tried to further simplify the mass of information flying about in her brain. In order to ensure consistency in representing the symbols, there was a rather complex set of instructions using terminology such as earthline, skyline, ascender and descender lines, composition square and so on. Kit tried to think of it along the lines of an old-fashioned learning-to-write book in which the child (in this case Kit) is taught to place each letter correctly between the upper and lower lines and the middle guiding line thus:

----------- Sky line-------------

....

----------- Earth line-----------

If you are old enough you will probably remember such practice books well. Add the idea of a regular-sized square to 'house' each symbol, with an extra line above for the symbol to indicate a part of speech e.g.

past	future	present	adverb
)	(	)(	V/\

and it begins to make sense. So here are some of the words which we first put on Harriet's personalised word chart. It may well be that Charles Bliss' spirit would have been unhappy, and the purists would no doubt hold up their hands in horror, but Kit made sure that the proportions remained constant, so that over the years the size of the symbol was reduced as would normally be the case for print size for children. We didn't have the luxury of time and needed to learn and adapt as we went along.

The first word chart was a large piece of sugar paper (rough paper used for children to paint on) cut to fit the wheelchair tray. Above each symbol was the written word:

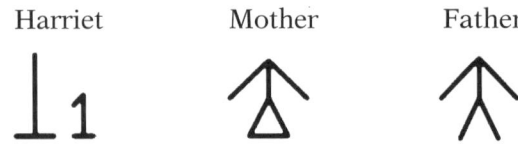

Harriet   Mother   Father

The symbol for person I with the number one 1 for I or me. On her chart we added an H for Harriet's name. We all called her 'aitch' a great deal of the time, 'Harriet' having proved difficult for some of her young friends to pronounce.

The words 'mother' and 'father' are made up of the symbol for woman or man, with a symbol above it to indicate the shelter or protection of belonging. (Kit's explanation, not necessarily the official one.)

Yes   No

$+!!$ $-!!$

– positive and negative symbols. We added traffic light
colours green and red to the appropriate word.

Other words we wanted H to have at her fingertips (or fist, to be more accurate) were some that allowed her to tell us how she was feeling, or what she wanted to do. The heart shaped symbol is used to indicate feeling, an arrow up or down shows good or bad feeling.

Happy   Sad

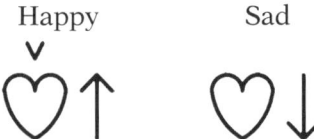

Combinations of signs and symbols can be arranged to make new words. Of course for Harriet the grammatical symbols for verb, adjective or adverb meant nothing at first, but as the number of words she knew grew so we introduced some of these symbols.

Other basic words on her early charts were:

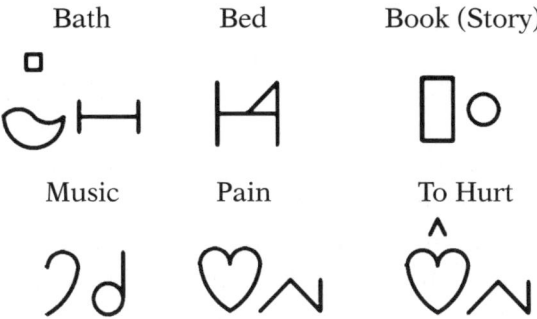

Two other words which we felt important and were combinations of symbols intended to allow H to express dislike or disapproval:

Rubbish

If you look at the different parts of the symbol it shows something not wanted put in the bin = rubbish.

Boring

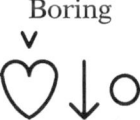

Similarly something that was said that is not liked = boring.

Rubbish became a very useful word. It could say "It's not fair!" or "don't patronise me" or "you're wrong" or even something less than complimentary depending on the context of the moment. We asked to visit the eye consultant again. Armed with her word chart Harriet had only one word of greeting to say: "Rubbish" – her fist went firmly onto the symbol.

She could have said hello, which was also one of the words currently being taught, but her choice expressed a lot of feeling in one word.

The consultant was duly impressed and Harriet's eyes were once again examined. This time it was declared that her sight was quite good, but some help with distance viewing was needed. Variable lenses were also prescribed to give her eyes protection against bright light.

Feeling vindicated, and it must be owned a trifle smug, Kit carried on with teaching Harriet as she thought best and gradually the store of words grew. By the time she was eleven years old Harriet had an impressive number of words at her command.

Her word chart now had a matrix of eight colour-coded pages. Seven of these were each divided into four columns made up of eight words. The eighth page was an alphabet page.

The colours were reproduced at the bottom of the chart and under them the numbers 1 to 8. Harriet could fist point to these blocks of colours and also to the numbers. Yes and No were at either side.

The process of identifying which word was being chosen had to be unvarying. It was always Question and Response. For example:

1. Question: Which colour page?
   Response: Yellow (fist pointing to the yellow block at the bottom of the chart).

2. Question: Which number column?
   Response: 3 (fist pointing to number at the bottom of the chart).

3. Question: Which number word?
   Response: 4.

So: Yellow. 3. 4. = Rubbish

The order was always the same namely: colour, column, word.

"Just imagine," Kit says "that before you utter every word during the day you first have to run up and down a flight of stairs carrying a heavy weight. You must do this not once, not twice, but three times for every single word. You will now have some understanding of how difficult it was for Harriet to make her arm move to pick a word from her chart."

In conjunction with the word chart, a special computer keyboard and programme of symbols was a useful teaching aid. The keyboard could be divided into spaces which could accommodate a pointing fist. Overlays were placed on the keyboard to allow Harriet to produce her written work. We could also test her knowledge by either asking her to correctly identify a symbol or word.

Here is an overlay from 1986 which Harriet was able to answer a question about who she had seen and where, or show that she could understand and recognise the symbol for friends.

school	hospital	I/me
⌂⏃⌂	⌂❕	⊥1
boy	girl	(to) see
⚨	⚨	∧ ⊙
the	park	with
╱	⚲⏄	✚
friends	car	aunt
⊥♡+!	⚙	△2⏄

Then on 27 June the entry in her daybook reads: "I with Mummy went to school to see girls. My friends."

A conversation with Daddy:

"Hello." (to Daddy)
"Happy, happy kiss." (Q. What about the kiss?)
"I want." (Q. Who do you want the kiss from?)
"Daddy." (Happy kisses given)
"Thank you."

On Monday, 24 November, after coming home from her friend Gareth's birthday party, when asked "which did you like the best, the food, the games, or the cuddle with Gareth in the chair?" Her reply is quite definite "chair".

Another entry shows her pleasure at getting some mail:

"Some letters for me. Liked letters."

The word order is often uncertain, sometimes she signals what she wants to talk about with a keyword such as "Happy" or after a day spent at Rookwood Hospital being fitted for a new seating mould:

"Chair – say how much liked."

The great difficulty in making her arm work to fist point accurately led to a rather telegraphic form of communication when she used as few words as possible to make her meaning clear. This often gives poignancy to her daily record, evoking memories of both joyful and sad times.

On a visit to the Blackburn family, everyone sat around the long table, Jo's children Katie, Sarah, Oliver and Edward and two friends of theirs all eating toasted hot cross buns (it was Easter time) except for H who was having her 'tea' of liquid balanced feed via her nasal gastric tube. There were ten of us sitting around the table, having much talk and fun, with Harriet watching and joining in the laughter. Later on, Kit asked her "What did you think of the visit to Jo's today?"

"Think. How laughed," was Harriet's reply, neatly capturing the essence of the entire afternoon.

When in 1989 John took early retirement in order to help at home Harriet was very pleased and said that she was "Happy. Daddy will be (at) home to give me kisses."

A PAGE FROM HARRIET'S WORD CHART

	1	2	3	4
1	GOOD	HAPPY	SAD	EASY
2	UPSET	FUNNY	NEW	DIFFICULT
3	BIRTHDAY	HOLIDAY	LETTER	OLD
4	CAR	STORY	RUBBISH	EXCITED
5	HOT	COLD	PAIN	WITH
6	THIRSTY	HUNGRY	TIRED	BETTER
7	PLEASE	THANK YOU	HELLO	MISTAKE
8	ANGRY	SICK	GOODBYE	DEAR

CHAPTER 7

Of Matters Spiritual

'Strength for today
and bright hope for tomorrow.'
T O Chisholm (1866–1960) – 'Great is Thy Faithfulness'

WE KNEW HOW imperfect and clumsy our efforts were to allow H to express herself. How conscious we were of the intelligence locked inside this body of hers; a body whose motor abilities were barely functioning because of implacable degeneration taking place in her brainstem. It was one of the most difficult aspects for us to accommodate emotionally. We take what comfort we can from the fact that, whatever its shortcomings, the system we had devised allowed H to share with us not only pleasure but some of her pain and fears.

Harriet had always found sleeping for any length of time at night difficult. Night sweats and painful joints from the Leigh's disease, together with an increasingly severe kyphosis and scoliosis of her spine (becoming both bowed and curved), made it hard for her to rest comfortably. But, during her ninth year, another worry surfaced and eventually we were able to discover what was troubling her.

Increasingly she was recording feeling tired and having a pain in her head. Sometimes she was unable to say what was wrong. On 14 September, in answer to the question, "Why do you cry so?" she replies "do not know. You have to love me."

During August matters began to crystallise. Cousin Susan had died rather unexpectedly and Kit was greatly upset, especially as her efforts to attend the funeral had been thwarted by a rail crash which made the journey to Cornwall impossible. On the eleventh of the month Harriet tells us that "Church was interesting. You are to understand cousin S came to Jesus." On 28 August she was "Feeling sad," Why? we asked. "To lie down, I feeling will know my deth [sic, using the alphabet card]." Further questioning helped to make it clear. Variously we read:

"Jesus helps my sad feeling."
"Am I sick?"
"My sad feeling Jesus will understand."

On 19 September once again:

"Upset. Difficult Mummy to say why. Death."

We realised that H was becoming aware that her illness was terminal and that she was afraid that she might die in her sleep, which was why she had become more upset and reluctant at bedtime. Her body was obviously becoming more tired and she was finding it difficult to cope with infections and pain.

During this time the Reverend Kelvin Richards gave her and us great support. Each week, when everyone was well, he would visit and talk to Harriet. Sometimes he would play a game of Connect 4 with her. Harriet felt that "Rev K is my friend." She asked him if after her death she would have a new body. He was able to reassure her that she would be free of all her earthly body's restrictions and during the course of their conversations she appeared to accept the fact of her illness and no longer seemed afraid of dying.

It would be less than honest to pretend that all callers offering spiritual guidance always received a calm and pleasant welcome. One morning in the time when Kit was coping on her own with both Harriet and granny, she was greeted by two ladies on the front doorstep who asked if she had five minutes "to talk about Jesus" with them. "Certainly" said Kit, who still had not been able to wash her face or comb her hair, "but what I need first is help to wash the bedroom carpet where Harriet vomited up her nasogastric tube earlier this morning, change the linen on her bed, clean the bath after her morning wash. Then my mother needs help to wash and dress and her bedroom needs attention. The kitchen floor needs cleaning and dirty dishes washing, I also have to get something to prepare for my mother's lunch and I'll have to go to the village shop for fresh vegetables. That's what I really need." The door was shut firmly on the two women. Five minutes later they were back again, offering to do all the tasks except helping granny to wash and dress. The offer was gratefully accepted. It would be good to be able to record that this was just the beginning. Sad to relate these two ladies did not come to offer help a second time.

John remembers a particular Sunday morning. He was entertaining Harriet who was in her standing frame. Kit was trying to oversee that and cook lunch simultaneously. Harriet was coughing and spluttering in her efforts to swallow and breathe. Kit opened the door to see a young man holding a leaflet about the Jehovah's Witnesses. "Ah," said Kit. "Just the person I need. In," she ordered. The poor chap was so surprised that he hurried after her as she went through to the dining area. There was Harriet with John. "Look," she demanded, as the young man followed. He looked. "Out" said Kit. The young man blenched and fled, without having said a word. Kit returned to the kitchen as Harriet and daddy fell silent as well. Eventually John ventured hesitantly to say, "Well Harriet, that was interesting wasn't it?" She coughed and spluttered in reply. Regardless of sect or religious persuasion, choose the wrong moment to pop your head above the parapet, and it would present an easy target for Kit in moments of stress. Andy, from the village church, presented himself early one evening. He knocked, and opened his mouth to speak as he proffered his collecting tin for a charity that we regularly supported. The door opened and Kit's snarled words "Not Now!" barely had time to get through the gap before the door slammed shut with a force that made the glass pane rattle. In all such encounters nobody seemed to bear any ill will and were remarkably understanding – though perhaps they did help to foster Kit's reputation as a 'hard woman'. The Rev K though, continued to call. Unassuming and gentle, his steadfast ministry was very important to us all.

It was he who suggested that, if Harriet wished, we could work towards her confirmation into the family of the Church – Harriet wanted to do this and with his regular visits, the Rev K took her through the full preparation course. Kit undertook to tackle the 'homework' with Harriet, using a variety of teaching aids and techniques. Once again a record of each step was recorded, filed and kept for the Rev K to see and approve as satisfactory. But, and it was a big but, Kit was unhappy at Harriet being confirmed as one of a group at a service where she would be unable to make her responses by speaking. If she was to be confirmed, it had to be properly done with Harriet able to make her responses to the bishop's questions to show that she understood what she was taking part in and what she was promising. Kelvin said that he would approach the bishop to see if he would agree to confirm her at home. He obviously made a good plea for her, and Dewi Bridges, Bishop of Swansea and Brecon, agreed to his request.

On 17 September 1991, Bishop Dewi arrived with Rev K to confirm Harriet. She had previously practised and written her responses with her computer overlays. Kit cut and pasted them onto individual pieces of card which were put in random order on the table in front of her. She would have to find the correct response to the bishop's questions which are the same as those asked of the child's godparents at the baptismal service. But this time it is those being confirmed who have to make the response for themselves. This was why Kit was so adamant that Harriet, having worked so hard to show that she understood the preparation over some three months, should also be able to show that she understood as well as the next ten or eleven year old the promises she was making.

The excitement was high when Bishop Dewi arrived. He changed into his vestments and came into the room where Harriet was ready and waiting. Two friends from the Church also came as a mini congregation. The bishop had previously been warned that he would need to sit facing Harriet and keep very still whilst she looked for her correct response from those on the table and fist pointed to it. The slightest distraction could send her into 'extension' or spastic movement, and she would have to start again.

Bishop Dewi had to sit himself on the low stool placed facing H. This stool had once belonged to Kit's great aunt Kitty, and had been brought to Llangynidr when her mother came to live with us. It is still in its original genuinely distressed green paint, narrow, unpadded and about six inches high, a very useful footstool. It was, and is, still known in our household as the 'stool of penitence' from the time when Harriet was using an ordinary low divan bed and we all had variously spent many night hours sitting beside her to watch over her breathing or to offer her comfort.

Arranging his robes the bishop asked his questions, held his arms wide and waited motionless as Harriet searched for and found her responses. The sacrament of wafer and wine was given by Bishop Dewi to Harriet and the mini congregation. Harriet had the smallest portion of wafer and a sip of wine from the special spoon that the bishop had brought, as she would be unable to sip from the chalice. As she accepted the wine and managed to swallow without too much splutter, H's face was almost radiant with pleasure and joy – a look probably mirrored on the face of everyone there.

The bishop gave Harriet a small book entitled *Giving Thanks, an aid to Worship at the Eucharist* and inscribed with his love. After this he and Rev K posed for a photograph with Harriet in the garden. The memory of her shining smile is indelible. On a later occasion Bishop Dewi said Harriet's confirmation was, for him, one of the most moving experiences of his episcopacy. He has also spoken of his pleasure on seeing Harriet's collage of Tenby when he came into the room as, prior to his elevation to the bishopric, he had been rector of St Mary's Church in Tenby.

At the time we had no idea that Bishop Dewi was not just a passing spiritual advisor and mentor, but had a further pivotal role to play in our lives. Harriet's confirmation was another stepping stone to the path that lay ahead for us both – a seminal moment in the later creation of Harriet's Trust.

CHAPTER 8

Tables and Topics

'The time has come the Walrus said
To talk of many things.'
Lewis Carroll (1832–98)

WHEN KIT'S MOTHER came to live with us, one of the things she brought with her was an unpolished wooden table with folding legs, rather like a trestle table. Kit remembered it from girlhood when her father used it as a marking table in his role as examiner and marker for the London University Board. Every summer several hundred exam scripts would arrive and father would be closeted away in the dining room, with the trestle table top covered with papers being marked. The table was already of venerable age when mother brought it to Llangynidr. It was probably nearly 50 years old then, having been acquired as army surplus at the end of the Second World War. We still have the table. It has found an honourable retirement in the Trust's office, where it is in daily use as a home for the printer and piles of brochures and booking forms for the four specially adapted houses established in Harriet's memory. However, for her, that table was an essential part of her school-room.

Harriet's schoolroom was the dining end of our living room, and the trestle table gave focus and display to the work we tackled to help increase her communication skills and learn as much as possible about her world. As ever the overriding aim was to make every day as interesting and joyful as we could. A topic approach seemed the most sensible and appropriate in view of her age and limited life expectancy.

So many topics to choose from, each one presenting opportunities for visits, art, music, stories, number work as well as writing and talking. A visit to the ballet to see *Coppelia* is one we remember well. The story, the music, artwork and the creation of a small 'book' about the ballet culminated in an outing to the New Theatre in Cardiff to see a live performance by the Northern Ballet Theatre in March 1989. Seated like royalty in one of the boxes, the auditorium packed with a 'holiday treat' audience of children and attending adults, Harriet greeted the by now familiar overture music with a cry of delighted recognition. The conductor, Brian Fieldhouse, looked up at her and gave a big smile before focusing back on the orchestra in the pit. Harriet settled, as did the whole audience, many of the children no doubt sharing for the first time that never failing frisson of excitement and expectation as the curtain rises on the magic that is the theatre.

Anything and everything was fair game for the table. Birthdays, the seasons, the weather, the countryside around us; the displays came and went in unbroken procession. During her short life Harriet had two carers, young women who came in each weekday to help look after her. Liz Jones came first and soon showed that she had a store of creative ability and enjoyed the many activities which filled our days. A memorable display featured a birthday cake with marzipan flowers to reproduce the bright flower bed in our small back garden. The real flowers picked from the garden filled the table top in multicoloured arrangements, together with some poetry and pictures.

When Liz left us, Gilly Lawrie came and within a very short time was assimilated into our family circle in a bond that has only strengthened as the years have passed. Tall, elegant, extremely talented, Gilly was also greatly caring and capable. Nothing was deemed impossible. We carried Harriet (or rather Gilly carried and mother puffed along behind) to the top of Mynydd Illytd to wonder at the views down to the valley below and across the majestic Pen-y-fan and the Brecon Beacon Mountains. We explored the Roman amphitheatre at Caerleon and gave baby goslings (borrowed for the day from Gilly's father) their first swim in Harriet's specially purchased hydraulic bath. Like naughty children we laughed with Harriet at their antics, and said "don't tell Social Services"! We went on the train to Hereford while Gilly drove Harriet's car to meet us at the station there before going to choose new clothes in the wheelchair-friendly shopping precinct. This was rounded off with a picnic in the park by the river.

All these were very ordinary activities but big achievements for a child as frail as Harriet. It was Gilly's infectious energy and enthusiasm which helped carry us along. Her ability to create almost any shape with a pair of scissors and some craft paper was fully extended and nurtured by Kit. Every day that Harriet was well was filled with activities, when she was not able to be up and about we read stories to her or played her favourite music. Television could be a problem as fits would be induced by any flickering light, and so, was more a treat for better days.

Two pieces of work that we tackled, with Gilly's skilful scissor work to the fore, are especially memorable and important in our recollections of Harriet's life.

Each 'term' we would choose one major piece of craftwork to centre round a current topic. When Harriet was nine years old we read the children's story *A Stitch in Time* by Penelope Lively. It tells the story of an only child, Maria, and what happens when she goes with her parents to stay at a holiday house near Lyme Regis. Maria learns that a girl named Harriet Polstead lived in the house more than a hundred years earlier. She had started to sew a sampler and hand embroidered images of her house, dog and a holly tree. The tree was still standing in the garden of the house. But the sampler had been left to her sister Susan to finish. Maria knew that she wanted to find out the reason why Harriet Polstead had left the sampler unfinished, and also why there were no photographs of the young girl in the old photograph album in the house. If you want to know how the story unfolds and ends you must read it for yourself, but as the story reads:

> Places are like clocks thought Maria. They've got all the time in them there's ever been, everything that's happened hidden in them, like you find the fossils if you break the rock.

Penelope Lively – *A Stitch in Time*

Our Harriet was enthralled by the story about her namesake, and so we made our own sampler. The alphabet and numerals one to nine were obligatory. In addition she chose to put pictures of our house, her three cats, her wheelchair, the adapted car, the canal, the mountains and swans, for being at home. A castle, sea birds and boats for holiday times. All these were chosen using word chart and alphabet card and took some considerable time. Each word necessitated at the very least three arm movements, and often considerably more. There were many times when we wished that Harriet had better control of her response times and finer accuracy, but she battled on.

Gilly cut out all the shapes ready for use. The craft 'moss-crepe' paper had the texture and appearance of material which echoed embroidery. With her word chart and computer overlay, Harriet composed her own quotation or text rather than choose the traditional Biblical one. "Time can come like a wind" she wrote. Words which echoed the story we had been reading. The computer printout was enlarged on a copier so that the letters no longer looked so 'print-like'. That was stage one.

Next we prepared the base on which to mount the work. We visited the craft shop to choose some embroidery canvas which was then stretched over the thin plywood baseboard. A smaller scale mock-up was prepared so that Harriet could fist-point to show where her various picture items were to be placed on the full-sized board. The alphabet letters and the numerals she had to sort in order, again by fist-pointing. Each item had to be fixed in place. Clutching a glue stick in her fist, Harriet laboriously smeared the adhesive onto the paper backing of the cut-out shape and Gilly helped her to press it onto the board. The finishing touches, her name Harriet Davis, 1989, 9 years, were spelt out using her word chart.

We felt that such an achievement for us all deserved to be preserved by being framed. Today it hangs beside two samplers inherited from Kit's maternal grandmother. 'Watch and Pray' admonishes one, 'The Lord will Provide' promises the second. Harriet's bright multicoloured design with its images of things beloved by her reminds us that 'Time can come like a wind' and that the hold on life that we have is at best tenuous and we may be blown off course as easily as if by a gust of wind.

And what was the second piece of work which is still evergreen in our memories? Strangely, it too was about the passage of time. The passage of a year. The same learning processes, learning the names of the twelve months, the days and weeks, all were part of a themed term's work. The main piece of craft work was to produce a calendar book. Not with all the days and weeks for each month, but an appropriate illustration and caption or sentence for each picture. The picture for the month of May is of a single red flower and leaf like a field poppy. Underneath are the lines:

Happy Flower
I kiss with
My red paint

But there is one month that is important and its illustration and caption known now to many more than just the family circle. The picture for the month of August repeats some of the images on the sampler. There are seagulls and the castle, only this time there are sandcastles on the beach with a bucket and spade nearby and the sea in the background. A seaside picture, with the caption:

I like to know everyone (to) have a holiday.

And there it was. A grain of sand lodges inside the oyster and eventually a pearl is formed; that small wish somehow lodged in our subconscious minds, until some three or four years later it surfaced, not a pearl, but a path we had to follow. It became the cornerstone upon which Harriet's Trust was founded.

CHAPTER 9

High Days and Holidays

'Tell me, my dear, whose voice you hear?
It is the sea, the sea...'
Charles Causley (1917–2003) – 'Tell me, Tell me, Sarah Jane'

ON THE WAY to the sea, the mountains of Breconshire behind us, we sang with gusto the chorus of the old music hall song:

Oh! I do like to be beside the seaside
I do like to be beside the sea
I do like to stroll upon the Prom, Prom, Prom,
Where the brass bands play
Tiddely om pom pom!

It became part of the holiday ritual as we neared Tenby and caught our first glimpse of the sea before driving down the hill into town.

The first time that we took Harriet to the seaside, in 1986, we were full of apprehension. A colleague of John's had a holiday bungalow on a small estate on the edge of Tenby. She very generously told us that we could use it free of charge if we wanted to try to take Harriet to the sea. Leaving Harriet with Liz for a few hours, we drove down to look at the bungalow and the beaches. As we stood at the end of the prom and looked along the long sandy South Beach, Kit breathed in deeply and said "If I can't have west Cornwall, then this will do."

We decided that three days would be manageable. Liz, Harriet's care assistant, offered to come with us, and her young daughter Katy came too. We had no adapted car then and Mike Chamberlain from Crickhowell volunteered to drive down with his minibus to spread the load a bit. The day of departure came; everything to be taken with us was laid out and John groaned "It will never all fit in." This also became part of the holiday ritual. Packing the car to go on the Tenby holiday or getting ready to return home, the familiar wail would be heard, "It will never all fit in." Portable suction machine, oxygen cylinder, medicines, feeds, shallow Sunflower bath to fit over the top of a normal bath (absolutely true), large inflatable physiotherapy ball over which we could drape Harriet for a daily postural drainage session – the list was long and most of the items bulky. However, everything did fit in. In all our years of Tenby holidaying, nothing was ever knowingly left behind because it would not fit in. When the adapted vehicle arrived, Harriet's wheelchair could be loaded straight in up the ramp and locked into position. Last minute packing was stowed all around her. Ill-advised spur of the moment purchases, usually plants quite unsuitable for the harsher Breconshire winter climate, would have to be balanced on knees or between feet. "There," we would chorus, peering through the foliage, "It's all fitted in. No need to fret John."

The few days in Tenby convinced us that holidays by the sea were possible as long as Harriet was free from chest infection or other temporary setback. On each future holiday Dr Cavenagh undertook to issue a 'Fit to Travel' certificate before our leaving home. He also phoned the surgery in Tenby and warned of our visit in case we had need of medical help during our stay. We must have achieved the status of a myth with them, as such help was never needed. Harriet used to send picture postcards to Dr Cavenagh with the message "Chest better because of sea air".

The following year we tried a house near Manorbier and auntie Joan, Kit's sister, came down to help. We also stayed in a large farmhouse at Garron Pill on the River Cleddau which was big enough for auntie Joan and uncle Arthur as well, to help with the chores. But as lovely as they were and as much as we went out exploring the beaches, something was lacking. Was it because at home we lived in a quiet corner of a small rural village? Not enough contrast perhaps? Looking through the book of holiday houses for rental, we spotted one right on Pier Hill in Tenby Harbour. Large enough to sleep nine or ten people and as close to the beach and harbour as we could wish. We decided to spend an extra week away and try it out. If it wasn't suitable, at least we would have had one good week beforehand we reasoned. The harbour and the small sandy beach there were already favourite places, with plenty of activity for Harriet to watch. We went to Lower Albion for that trial week and unwittingly the future course of our lives was laid down.

There were, of course, no special facilities for a disabled child there. The kitchen was on the ground floor, but the sitting room, bedrooms and bathroom were all on the second level. We had to manhandle the wheelchair down a steep step into the house and carry H upstairs. In a twin-bedded room we pushed the beds together so that Harriet could lie in the middle and not be at risk of falling onto the floor. Not ideal by any means, but, the house was big enough for all our needs and also to have family and friends to help. The large table in the kitchen became the focal point for meals and talk about the day. Harriet could be included in the gathering. Upstairs the windows looked out on all the harbour activity, boats coming and going to Caldey Island, holidaymakers, the tide's ebb and flow, gulls screaming in the morning, always something happening.

After her holiday in June 1988 Harriet said that the most interesting thing about the week had been "the harbour". We have a snapshot, one of many, of her sitting there on the sand in the sunshine with auntie Joan holding her from behind, the water lapping around them, laughing up at her father, her pleasure and happiness quite apparent. In 1989 we all remember how hot the summer was. This time we had a house full. Cousins Christine and Alan from Cornwall, auntie Joan and Uncle Arthur, John and Angela McFall with their sons David and Gethyn, two of Harriet's beloved 'best boys'. Long days of sun were spent on the harbour beach. The cars were parked on arrival and only moved again on the day of departure.

That year became the year of sandcastle making. During the week under John's organizational skills, ambitions of size and design grew apace. But each day, as the tide came in, even more fun was had splashing about and jumping on the rapidly vanishing castle walls. Harriet couldn't jump or dig, but she was in the midst of the action and included by all the children. Going along the North Walk above the North Beach, David would urge Harriet to see how many toes she could run over, and they would encourage her to take off down the beach towards the sea. "Next year" Gethyn said, "I'll be old enough to go for the papers by myself." Memories of childhood holidays are absorbed and as with all experiences, become part of who we are. Sixteen years on, visiting Tenby Harbour with his parents as a young adult, Gethyn reportedly got to his feet saying "I'm going to make a sandcastle J D would be proud of." J D, that is John, could ask for no better endorsement.

During those few brief years of holidays in the house on Pier Hill the daily round of activities were very ordinary. The routine of postural drainage to help keep H's chest clear, medication and liquid feeds required that strict timekeeping had to be kept. Otherwise we did what any other family on a self-catering holiday does. We walked through Castle Square behind Pier Hill, past Laxton House where the old seabaths were once a popular venue for visiting gentry. We stopped to look at the Greek inscription above the door and learnt the translation: "The sea washes away man's ills." We walked the paths around Castle Hill which rises above the harbour and gives far-reaching views across the bay with sandy beaches nearby, Caldey Island ahead and the coastline stretching away.

On a fine day the coast of the Gower or Lundy Island, off the Devon coast, can be seen. One of the steep paths up to the top of Castle Hill passes a mosaic mural of words and images of the sea. Kit would take Harriet to look closely at the nine panels depicting the castle ruins on the hill, with the blues and greens of the sea stretching across with white waves and sea birds. She would read the words above each panel to Harriet. Greek, Welsh, Latin, English – all of them about the sea. Words from Psalm 95: "The sea is His and He made it"; Xenophon's words, in Greek and English: "The sea. The sea." So simple, yet so evocative. Best known, for Harriet were lines of the American poet Emily Dickenson:

> I started early, took my dog
> And visited the sea,
> The mermaids in the basement
> Came out to look at me.

Tenby Museum was then, sadly, not very accessible for Harriet's wheelchair, but a visit to the monument of Albert, Queen Victoria's consort, with the remains of the old fort dominating the summit of the hill, was another part of the holiday ritual. The steep path back down to the bandstand needed great care with the wheelchair but once safely down we might go to the shops to buy small presents to take back to friends at home. The fudge shop was always popular.

The Lifeboat Station was just around the corner from Castle Square, but unfortunately inaccessible to wheelchairs. Today, a grand new housing for the boat is approached by a level walkway giving easy access to the shop and the gallery overlooking the boat when it is not at sea or out on a 'shout'. However when the maroons were fired to call the lifeboatmen to duty, we could not avoid hearing them – and the windows of the house would rattle. The children would count to see if the call was for the inshore boat or for the all-weather seagoing, Tyne Class, Sir Galahad. Then we would all keep alert to see when the boat returned to base. Even greater excitement if the return came after dark when, by the lights in the harbour, the children watched the activity from the windows of the house. One morning we were all sitting around the breakfast table making plans for the day ahead when Alan Thomas, the lifeboat coxswain, knocked at the door. "We're having a practice run" he said, "launch in about five minutes if you want to watch." We bundled Harriet in a blanket and carried her out with the boys to the harbour wall where we could see the lifeboat house and slip clearly. We gave a cheer as the boat came down the slip sending up a big wave and spray as it hit the water. A very good start to the day.

There was only one seaside activity left that Kit wanted Harriet to have a chance to experience – a trip on the water. We had watched the small boats coming and going taking visitors across to Caldey Island or around the bay, or mackerel fishing. We didn't feel confident enough to go to Caldey and land; the electric wheelchair was heavy and we would need, as ever, the suction machine and portable oxygen cylinder. But a trip just around the island when we might see seals on the rocks, and gannets and cormorants, on the high cliff – that was a possibility. We wrapped H up well and a young boatman carried her easily down the harbour steps onto one of the boats. We held her on our laps, supporting her body with ours. Once again she was able to be part of a very ordinary holiday event and proved to be a good sailor, obviously interested and enjoying every moment.

One outing we did take from Tenby was to the old Bishop's Palace at Lamphey where, the few ruined walls that remain, in some way sparked Harriet's interest in castles and ancient monuments.

The sun didn't shine everyday on every holiday; rain and wind on mid-summer's day 1990. The daybook records that it rained and rained all day. Harriet wants to know, "Can have game, please?" The rainy days did not spoil the memories of the week, and back home again she says "Holiday with friends I loved."

The following year, on our return to Lower Albion on 8 June, she tells us "Happy to come here. I remember my bedroom." It was raining when we arrived and again on Tuesday, 11 June it was windy, with rain. Nonetheless H wanted to send her usual postcard to Dr Sandy because she felt that "Chest pretty good. Better because of the sea." On the Friday of that week, the weather was cool and windy but at least the rain had eased. A trip to Pendine sands was mooted. This is where, famously, Donald Campbell broke the land-speed record in his Bluebird car. Harriet, not to be bested, put the wheelchair which had replaced her outgrown Turbo through its paces. "New chair drove. Weather windy. Thank you chair, interesting to have you to drive." Kit recorded that Harriet wore: winter trousers, tights, coat, hat, scarf, gloves and wheelchair cover for the run along the hard sands. All accompanying adults were similarly well-protected against the cold wind. High summer indeed.

The children were always loath to leave when the holiday was over. Angela McFall remembers Harriet vomiting up her nasogastric tube about ten minutes before departure. Everything had to be put on hold until the tube was replaced, with Harriet determined to make it as difficult as possible.

"You wouldn't believe it" laughed Angela, "How could she do that deliberately?"

"More easily than you imagine," was Kit's opinion.

Once back home post-holiday blues would descend and then, just before Christmas, Harriet would start to ask if her father had booked the holiday house and sent the money for the chosen weeks.

In October 1991 we all went for our autumn seaside holiday. Kit was finding it evermore difficult to manage to wash and dress H on an ordinary bed. Bathing was no longer possible. Harriet was now nearly as tall as Kit and it was dangerous to try and lower her into an ordinary bath. It would be only too easy to drop her and Kit's back was already damaged from lifting and carrying over the years. At the back of her mind was the fear that she would not be able to continue indefinitely with arrangements as they were at present.

But, once back home, the holiday for 1992 was booked as usual. Just after Christmas Harriet became unwell with a chest infection. A short stay in hospital seemed, despite Kit's forebodings, to set things right. Then, without warning, the day before we were due to return home, the plateau of Leigh's disease that Harriet had been on, came to an abrupt end. Without fuss she slipped over the precipice, and within two days it was finished. We returned home to the silence and the grief and to try to make sense of all that had happened in the previous twelve years.

Interlude
by Rose Hopkins

I first met Harriet when she came to the children's ward aged just ten months with Kit and Granny Roberts. Little did I know then that this little child with the very big name, Miss Harriet Catherine Frances Davis, would become a very large and special part of my life. That visit became the first of many for Harriet, Kit and John – from then on life changed for them.

I still remember how proud I felt when Kit asked me if I would consider helping to look after H at home for a few hours each week. From then on we became firm friends, which we still are today. A few weeks later I began to make my visits to 1 Bryncelyn Way, to help look after Harriet and support Kit and John in any way necessary. I have many wonderful memories of 'H' and these are just a few.

The pleasure she got sitting with me watching some of her favourite TV programmes for fifteen minutes after lunch, playing her musical instruments whilst singing along to an LP of Sally Army music, making a lot of noise and laughing. She also enjoyed being read to from her favourite books, moulding play-dough and painting. I remember the faces she pulled when having yoghurt for dessert – we both hated yoghurt! The way she always coughed and vomited when birthday candles smoke rose into the air at a party!

Not so happy memories are Harriet being ill and having to spend time back on the children's ward; of her regularly coughing up her 'NG' tube and the numerous attempts to replace it by Kit or myself whilst she patiently sat smiling throughout. She was always smiling even when she was ill and obviously feeling ghastly. She never fussed. Life became an emotional rollercoaster for us all, being happy when she was well and worried and concerned when she wasn't. Harriet however, just kept bouncing back and kept on smiling while we just took one day at a time.

As she grew and was able to communicate using her word chart, her true personality shone through. As soon as she learned how to use it she never stopped talking, she loved using it. Walking up the drive when I visited, I would see Harriet sitting with Kit waving and smiling. Once inside we would kiss and hug, then immediately after, we had to chat, using the word chart she began saying: "Hello Auntie Rose, kiss." Followed by "Rubbish" and great laughter before moving on to the news and gossip of what had happened since my last visit.

Seeing Harriet grow and develop beyond everyone's expectations was wonderful. The credit for this can only be taken by Kit and John. They never gave up even though the diagnosis of her illness was poor and life limiting. They stayed positive throughout and I have nothing but the greatest admiration for them both. Harriet could not have had more wonderful parents.

I loved Harriet very much; she was a beautiful child, both inside and out. She touched the hearts of everyone she met; she was an inspiration to us all. It was both a privilege and a pleasure to have been able to play a small part in her life; a life, although short, was filled with love, laughter and happiness. She will never be forgotten, but remembered with love and affection always.

Interlude
by Alva Corbett

I came into Harriet's life when she was just two and a half years old. I had applied for a job as a night nurse in the local community hospital which I did not get but, instead, was offered a post in the community, to sit with a severely handicapped child two nights a week to give her parents a break. The Health Board had already placed a nurse in the home on a temporary basis. According to the senior nurse who interviewed me, it would probably be a short-term post as the child had a very poor prognosis – little did I know that my 'temporary contract' would last for eight and a half years.

The first time I saw Harriet she was sound asleep in bed. Linda, the temporary nurse was on duty, I was to stay with her for a few hours to learn the ropes. I could not believe that this beautiful little girl could possibly have anything wrong with her. The only clue was a tiny nasogastric (NG) tube protruding from her nostril, taped to her cheek and disappearing behind her ear. I stayed until about three in the morning with Linda, and then quietly let myself out of the front door. Harriet still had not met her night nurse. Next time I would be flying solo. I had met her parents, Kit and John, on arrival. As it turns out John knew my husband. John was the local Community Development Officer and he and Jeremy had met through work.

We all settled into a routine. I would turn up at 9.30 p.m. on two mutually agreed nights of the week. Harriet would be tucked up asleep in bed. She shared a bedroom with her parents, sleeping in a single bed beside theirs. The nights I was there Kit and John moved into the spare room. We would all have a cup of coffee and hear each others news. I would then settle into my armchair at the foot of Harriet's bed and prepare to read, sew or knit the night away. Kit and John would put their head around the door about 11 p.m. to say goodnight and silence would descend on the house. One of the cats might visit and snuggle down to sleep on a bed. I would turn Harriet every two hours and change her nappy if need be. Kit would appear around 7.30 a.m. with cups of tea for us all by which time Harriet would usually be awake. She would give Harriet her tea down the NG tube. I would report on our night and we would usually chat until eight when I went home. That was on a good night.

Harriet was prone to chest infections. Any visitor with even a hint of a sniffle was discouraged, but it was inevitable that some viruses would invade. Harriet could become quite poorly very quickly and often needed hospitalisation. She was well known in the children's ward in Abergavenny Hospital. Moreover, the family built up a very special relationship with their GP, Dr Sandy Cavenagh. Harriet loved him, she knew him as Uncle Sandy. He never did 'a home visit' but 'swerved by'. He went on to become president of the Trust, and remains a loyal friend to this day.

Harriet was unable to speak but Kit had found a way to release her from her silent world by teaching her to communicate by pointing to letters on a chart. Harriet sat on her mother's knee facing outwards with Kit supporting and holding her head steady. The two moved as one. We all adopted the same stance when we were holding Harriet. She had just enough power in her right hand, if supported, to direct her fist to point at each letter. This method of communication was used through the day but we didn't usually have to employ it at night. However, I found that over the years I got so tuned in to this little girl's every breath and movement that they were as familiar as my own.

Some nights Harriet could just be wakeful. I would crouch down beside her on a little footstool and hold her hand or stroke her hair. She would just watch me smiling, eventually falling asleep. I too could nod off, and on waking find that I had completely seized up too, bent in two unable to move. Afraid of disturbing my little sleeping beauty I would painfully and slowly crawl on all fours back to my chair to try to straighten my aching back.

On the nights she was poorly she sometimes struggled to keep her usual good humour, becoming frustrated and on occasions crying. She needed extra fluids via the NG tube. Unfortunately, the tube could often be coughed up in a fit of coughing, requiring replacing, usually with the aid of a suction machine. All this must have been so distressing for a little girl but she bore it all with such stoicism. As you can imagine, this caused quite a racket. The cat usually fled the scene but Kit never interfered unless I asked her. I hated disturbing her but there were times when I just had to have her help to settle Harriet.

Kit's mother was living with the family in a newly-built extension but sadly her health deteriorated and Kit was now nursing her as well.

As the story of the two ladies who arrived on the doorstep one morning just after I had left, wanting to talk about Jesus shows, Kit could be a formidable lady. She was like a lioness fighting for her cub. I told her on many an occasion that I was glad I was in her gang. Life seemed to be an endless battle to receive the help that was needed for Harriet.

Many people did not believe that Harriet had the intellect to be able to understand the spoken word and, in turn, be able to communicate. This was particularly upsetting as Kit had been a teacher of children with learning difficulties. Anyone who had anything to do with Harriet could clearly see that she was a very bright child whose life was completely enhanced by her mother's teaching.

No challenge was too great. The Royal Air Force was brought to task. We have all experienced that heart-stopping moment of fear when a low-flying jet fighter plane flies overhead and, at this time, mid Wales was a favourite area for training flights at night as well as by day. But for Harriet, a sudden noise like that could and did pre-empt a fit. So Kit phoned and wrote to the Air Ministry explaining the situation and was eventually visited by a very nice officer who was completely charmed by Harriet's smile and agreed that in future planes flying over the Davis household would restrict their speed! It was very noticeable thereafter that the planes were indeed slower, I'm sure if the pilot could have tooted a horn he would have done!

Life went on. Kit's mother sadly died. Relatives came and went, another stray cat was taken in and Kit and John took on even more work. They had decided to open a second-hand charity shop in Brecon to raise money for the charity Research into Metabolic Diseases in Children (RMDC). This is where John's talents were put to good use. He too was a born organizer, and had valuable experience and knowledge of applying for grants.

Now their evenings were taken up with sorting out donated clothes bags and ironing garments ready for the shop. Often, if Harriet was having a good night, I spent many hours ironing too. I also, on occasions, looked after Harriet during the day – sometimes just to let Kit and John have a day in the garden or just a much needed break. The reality was that there were very few people who could do this. There was either Harriet's much loved and trusted day carer Gilly, Rose or me. And even then it was not always easy to persuade Kit to have a break.

Harriet was now growing quite tall and, of course, heavier. This was taking its toll on Kit's health. She was developing pains in her joints. It eventually was decided to renovate granny's old rooms downstairs for Harriet. These were converted into a fantastic bathroom with equipment for disabled use and the bedroom was beautifully decorated by John. Kit moved down to share with Harriet and my old armchair came too.

As you can see, this nursing post was a little out of the ordinary. Anyone who became involved with the family developed a deep sense of loyalty and for me a great admiration and awe at what they had achieved, not to mention an immense love for my little patient. When a household settles at the day's end it is a very private time and I always felt it a great privilege to be present year in and year out. I was there through the best of times but also the worst of times.

When Harriet died in hospital she was brought home and laid in her own little bed. I went to see her and sat by her bed, held her hand and stroked her hair. There was just her and me, one last time.

Harriet's short life was full of difficulties, but what a legacy she has left. Inspired by Harriet's wish for everyone to have a family holiday like she did, her parents have established the Harriet Davis Trust providing holiday homes for families with disabled children.

Harriet filled eight-and-a-half-years of my life and the life of my family but she will be in my heart forever. It's been a privilege to have been part of this tale of heartbreak, human strength and love.

CHAPTER 10

And so it begins

'The house is great; it enabled us to take a holiday at the seaside, which would not have been possible otherwise. Are these houses truly unique? Certainly we have found nothing elsewhere equipped to this standard.'

Quote from a Visitors' Book

HARRIET DIED IN January 1992 and as we had previously, at her insistence, booked her favourite holiday house overlooking the harbour in Tenby, we decided that if we did not go for a holiday we would never go to Tenby again. So, with the friends who usually came with us, we went, knowing that we could always go home if it proved too much. However, it was very successful and the memories of Harriet's enjoyment of holidays by the sea helped the healing process for us. This experience has prompted us to offer, to families who have used one of the Trust's houses and whose children have died, to take up their holiday booking and all have found this to be of great benefit.

Whilst we were there we were touched by the sympathy of many local people who had seen us in previous years with Harriet, even those who had only seen her out and about in her wheelchair. Bing, who sold the tickets from the kiosk at the top of Pier Hill for the Caldey Island boats, enquired after 'the little girl' and shed a tear when told that she had died. Kit explained to Julie Schofield, who at that time lived in a small house on the harbour, that it would have been difficult to bring H on holiday much longer, as she was growing and it was not possible to look after her properly without all the special equipment that was needed. We had found that without the profiling bed, hydraulic bath and hoist, it was becoming very difficult to cope in a house that did not have these aids. By this time Harriet was almost as tall as Kit and trying to support her inert weight without aids was dangerous, especially going up and down stairs and lowering her into an ordinary bath. Dressing her on an ordinary bed was also placing great stress on Kit's back. It was during this conversation with Julie that Kit had one of those 'how do I know what I think until I hear what I say' moments. The seed planted in our subconscious mind by our experiences whilst Harriet was alive had become the pearl ready to see the light of day. Having met other families with disabled children, we thought that there might be a need for adapted accommodation. "What is needed is a house that is fully equipped with all the aids with which to care for a disabled child," she told Julie. Of course this was really Harriet's idea when she had 'said' that she thought everyone should have a holiday.

Immediately, Julie told Kit that Upper Albion, the property above the one we were staying in was for sale and that the owner, David Manby, of whom more later, was there. So we went to see him. At this point it is necessary to explain that the houses on Tenby harbour are divided rather eccentrically, and whilst Upper Albion is above Lower Albion suggesting a first floor flat, it is actually accessed directly from Castle Square that leads to the Lifeboat Station, so that the entrance is suitable for wheelchair users. As in Lower Albion the windows all overlook the harbour where something is always going on, be it tourists coming and going to Caldey Island, provisions, including cattle and machinery being loaded on the Caldey boat, fishing boats, yachts and motor boats and children digging in the sand. We know that many children enjoy, as Harriet did, watching the ever-changing scene. Charlie Crockford MBE, erstwhile mechanic of the Tenby lifeboat, described the view as the best in Tenby.

David, who we had never met before, was very welcoming and when Kit explained her idea he was immediately enthused and said, "We'll do it then."

It must be said that the house was not in the best condition and some of the arrangements somewhat strange to say the least. For example, the bath was semi-sunken and to get into it one had to turn sideways through a narrow archway and at the same time lower oneself precariously into the blue steel bath. We were rather flummoxed to see water running into the bath from its overflow and, after much investigation, discovered that the overflow from the toilet was routed to it. David, who was awarded an OBE for his work at the Agricultural Research Institute at Silsoe, was one of the great eccentrics and never threw anything away that he thought might be of the slightest use. There were three vacuum cleaners in the house, none of which worked, but David felt that he could make a workable one from them. In what had been a kitchen a rusting anchor lay at rest together with half-used tins of paint and other sundry nautical items. However, he undertook building projects that no one else would ever have contemplated and several otherwise derelict properties in Tenby were brought into use due to his ingenuity.

We really had no idea of the task that we had undertaken but, fortunately, our previous experiences had equipped us to a certain extent and of course Harriet's needs had provided us with some knowledge of the special equipment required. Building works were an unknown territory. It was clear to us that in order to be able to raise the money required to buy the property, adapt it, buy all the furnishing and equipment necessary, we would have to establish a charity. John, in his role as a Community Development Officer, had been responsible for advising groups and organizations on the availability of grants for community halls and sports facilities and had knowledge of what was required to achieve charitable status. With charitable status it would be possible to raise money from public donations, fund-raising events and applications to grant making bodies. We had to decide on the objects of the charity, who it was going to benefit, what should it be called and who we were going to ask to act as Trustees.

We finally hit upon the name and decided that it should reflect Harriet's wish. So the Trust became, *The Harriet Davis Seaside Holiday Trust for Disabled Children*, with the main objective of:

> To relieve disabled children and in particular: to purchase take on lease establish equip and maintain a property or properties in seaside holiday locations suitably constructed or adapted to enable disabled children their families or carers to enjoy the benefits of seaside holidays.

We appreciated that the Trust would need a patron with some gravitas and standing in the community. Diffidently, we approached Bishop Dewi Bridges who had confirmed H. After we had explained what we wanted to do he was kind enough to agree to become the patron of the Trust. A charitable trust can also have a president and vice-presidents in honorary positions to add to the standing of the charity. We asked Dr Sandy Cavenagh, a much-respected GP in Brecon and beloved by Harriet, to become the president. Maj. James More-Molyneux of Loseley Park and his wife Sue, together with David Mamby agreed to be vice-presidents. As Trustees we recruited those who had known Harriet. Jan Boreham, her physiotherapist, came on board and provided invaluable advice on the equipment required. Angela McFall, mother of two of H's best boys, Jo Blackburn, pre-school playgroups' organizer who we had first met at the hydrotherapy pool, Barrie Jones, a co-member of Brecon Lions' Club with John and Bryn Williams, secretary of the Brecon and Radnor Community Health Council of which John was chairman at that time, all agreed to act as Trustees.

We completed the documentation required by the Charity Commission who, with minor amendments, speedily approved the charity deed which John had written; this was a surprise as we had been warned by others that it would take some time.

At this time Harriet's computer was old and unsuitable for the task ahead; the internet was in its infancy and the National Lottery did not exist. Kit, having bought the large book about charitable trusts, began to research through it looking for any that included the needs of the disabled in their grant policy, and those which were not restricted in their geographical area of giving. A list was gradually assembled. Sitting at the dining table, back wedged against the radiator, she set about handwriting over 300 letters telling Harriet's story and our plans to enable other families with disabled children to have holidays together. The letters were posted in small batches. We felt as if we were following King David's advice in the book of Ecclesiastes, casting our bread upon the waters, although not with any firm expectation of a great return.

After a month David phoned to ask if we were going ahead with the project and when we said yes he promised to hold the house for us. All the fund-raising and the story of the charity shop deserve a chapter for themselves to give the full flavour of the fun and anguish. At this stage however, two things provided us with the encouragement to see the project through: firstly, the very generous support received from many kind individuals through donations and support of the fund-raising and, secondly, one morning after Kit had become despondent about our eventual success, a letter arrived from the Tudor Trust promising a grant of £25,000 and, whilst we were not permitted to mention the amount at that stage, we were able to mention the support of the Trust to other potential donors. Lift off! Eventually some £130,000 was raised, much of it whilst the adaptations to Upper Albion, which by this time was becoming known as 'Harriet's House', were being undertaken.

Over a century ago the property had been the Albion Hotel, an establishment that announced, by way of a plaque on the front wall, that '"concoctions" were available to "travellers" by steamers and the crews of trading craft and all users of the harbour'. The rivalry between the Barnstaple and Tenby fishing fleets often flared into fist-fights, and so, two bars were provided, hence Upper and Lower Albion. Also in Castle Square is Laston House which was built by Paxton in about 1810 to provide saltwater baths and refreshment rooms for the gentry. We were already familiar with the plaque on the wall of the house which claims, in Greek, that 'the sea washes away all man's ills'. Castle Square was also the scene of a rally by Mrs Pankhurst, leader of the women's suffrage movement. Tenby, of course, has a long history and is one of the few remaining medieval walled towns and was a very busy port with, among other things, a thriving wine trade with Brittany which encouraged smuggling.

Roger Toms of Barrington Builders was recommended by David to carry out the conversion of the property, and plans were drawn up by the Willis and Hole Partnership; these showed that the whole place needed gutting, especially so when it was discovered that the beams holding up the floor and which formed the ceiling of one of the houses below, were beginning to rot away. Rather than have all these replaced, which the owners of the other property were loath to consider, a new floor was 'hung' over the existing. This involved removing interior walls and two tons of quarry tiles from what was an old kitchen. At a meeting with Roger and David to discuss the cost of the new floor, Kit asked how much this would cost and after some considerable prompting Roger came up with a guesstimate of £5,000. We managed to mask our fears about raising the money and privately wondered what we had taken on. We were too far into the project to withdraw, so told him to carry on, and later David reduced his asking price for the house by the same amount. We only learnt some years later, after he had died, that David Manby had assured Roger Toms that he would underwrite his bill should we fail to raise enough. What a wonderful man he was, although his philosophy of life, that everything, however old or worn had its use, did cause us some problems. In the lounge there was an orange carpet that he wanted us to reuse, but when it was taken up it almost fell into pieces and it would not have fitted into the new configuration of the room. During the alterations David continued to be concerned about the fate of the carpet, having seen one rather like it in a skip in the town. After the opening of the house David asked what had become of it, and John assured him that it had gone to a good home. There was a similar problem with the blue bathroom suite and Roger had to put it into store for use in the future, where it may still be. Another of his concerns was an antique oak corner cupboard, but this remains in its original place in the living room and, appropriately, given the history of the house, is used to store all the drinking glasses.

On one memorable occasion David and John were to have a meal and discussion with Nick Hole, the architect, and met in Castle Square. David arrived in an old van saying that he had driven from Carmarthen without any lights and that the brakes were failing, however John was not to worry as the handbrake was working and he had been a rally driver. Alternative transport was quickly sought.

Under Roger's direction the workmen who he had recruited melded into a really great team and were strongly motivated by the idea of a holiday house for families with disabled children. They all worked hard for long hours to meet our deadline. Apart from the problem with the main floor there were other moments of difficulty and hilarity. The floor, in what was to be the 'special' bathroom, collapsed into the cellars beneath and the wall to the adjoining property moved alarmingly. A flight of narrow slippery steps leading down to the damp cellars was revealed underneath the floor, so too a short tunnel going a few feet under the square where stalactites had formed. It is easy to imagine these being used by smugglers when they extended further, possibly even to Castle beach. In Tenby High Street there is another tunnel that leads from what is now Boots, the chemist, to St Mary's Church opposite. It is reputed that Henry Tudor used this tunnel as an escape route after the battle of Tewkesbury, 1471.

Three bay windows overlooking the harbour side of the house all had to be replaced as the wood was rotten. These windows were a later alteration to the building and the Pembrokeshire Coast National Park would have preferred us to change them to the original sash windows, but accepted that they had become a feature of the property. Indeed they are part of the iconic view of Tenby Harbour and feature in many of the postcards, photographs and paintings of the harbour. Moreover, we considered that they enhanced the view from the house. Erecting scaffolding for this work presented a problem as Lower Albion was being let to visitors at this time, so, after doing some of the work it had to come down and then be put back up the following week. Unfortunately during this next 'window of opportunity' it rained, but eventually they were completed between the showers and Roger's team decided that the lead worker should be shut out on the scaffolding until he had finished the job.

Julie, from the house next to the Caldey Island stores on the pier, kept up a regular supply of cake and doughnuts for Roger's team, and we made frequent visits down from Brecon. The chaos of the early days of gutting the rooms, with walls, windows and floors being replaced, soon gave way to a more orderly progression of replacement and adaptation. Central heating was installed and the new 'special' bathroom began to take shape. The sewerage system that serves the harbour area is old and somewhat delicately temperamental in its operation, but we were assured that this extra bathroom would not cause an overload. Kit began the enjoyable part of choosing colours, furniture and fittings. We knew what basic special equipment would be needed and went to the National Association of Disability Exhibition (Nadex) to ensure that the equipment was as up to date as possible. Jan Boreham gave invaluable advice on what would be needed. We knew that we would be not be able to offer the ideal situation to everybody's needs, but hoped to find a good workable compromise for all. As it has transpired, something must have been done right because, in eighteen years of operation, only one family has ever found it to be unsuitable for their needs. Other families have been so impressed with what had been supplied that they have returned home to badger their local social services departments for some of the same. The equipment, of course, has been kept up to date, as necessary.

The bath was the easiest to decide upon. Harriet had been given a fine bath through the health and social services, funded with a legacy that was given with the wish that it be spent on some equipment for a child. The height was adjustable and the side opened down to enable easy transfer from wheelchair to bath and there was special quick drying cushioning as well as an adjustable headrest. A Kingcraft bath – very aptly named we thought. This was the same bath in which visiting baby goslings were given their first swim, much to Harriet's delight. She had loved her bath time when the house would be filled with exotic scents of oils and bubble baths. Lady's mantle and violet was a particularly lush combination. Our relationship with Social Services, shaky at the best of times, had taken a nosedive when Harriet died because of their initial handling of Gilly's contract of work and we knew that much returned equipment was left rusting in an old damp shed. Kit's reputation as a formidable and hard woman was firmly established, and nobody from the authorities showed any inclination to ask her for the return of the bath. We decided that if the bath was rehomed in Harriet's House, it would be well-used, appreciated and be in keeping with the wishes of the original donor.

The only stumbling block was how to get the bath to Tenby. Every village worthy of its name should have a village handyman – in Llangynidr this was Trevor Meredith, who dealt good humouredly with building, tiling, plumbing, plastering and small repairs of all types. He had helped us on a number of occasions, including the installation of the special bath in the new bathroom we created for Harriet. We knew that he had a flatbed truck and asked him if he would transport the bath to Tenby. He readily agreed and said that he and his labourer Sharkey, a young man of strength if not intellect, would go on a 'works outing' to the seaside. The bath was lashed onto the truck and off they went. We could picture it bouncing its way to its new home and hoped that it would arrive safely. On the way back Trevor and Sharkey stopped to refresh themselves at a convenient pub. Sharkey obviously entered whole-heartedly, if not wisely, into the outing spirit – equally obviously, he did not have a good head for alcohol and made some ill-judged remark about Trevor's building ability – along the lines of he couldn't build a brick house. Trevor took offence and by the time they arrived back in the village, Sharkey had been sacked. We felt rather responsible but eventually they made up their differences.

Harriet's House was now beginning to look less like a demolition site and more habitable. Curtains were being made, furniture ordered and the final painting and decorating started. Eventually all was assembled and the carpets were laid. Equipping the kitchen seemed to create a lengthy list of things to get: rather like moving house when the contents of the kitchen cupboards take longer to pack than almost anything else. Amongst many donations given were: a cupboard full of glassware from Julie on the harbour, a large pine dining table from the Tenby Brownie Pack, which they 'walked' through the town to take its place in the living room, and the Tenby and Saundersfoot Soroptimists paid for a beautiful specially commissioned pine dresser. We were overwhelmed by the generosity of so many people, numbers of whom were previously unknown to us.

We continued to journey back and forth from Llangynidr to Tenby. If the car had been a horse and cart, the horse would probably have found its own way home by the time the formal opening arrived. Before that day there were many important tasks which had to be juggled alongside the building works: printing brochures about the Trust, getting the first year's bookings from families, appointing someone to look after the house and help families to settle in on arrival at the harbour.

Again Kit sent letters, together with the brochures, in various directions: disability support organizations, social services departments and hospitals where the information could be passed on, day and boarding special needs schools were on the list. Nearer to home Jan Boreham spread the news amongst the families of children she saw as a paediatric physiotherapist and she also gave brochures to occupational therapists. John, in his role as honorary secretary of the Children's Centre at the Neville Hall Hospital, kept the staff there informed of our progress.

The ladies who helped in our charity shop in Brecon ensured that all the customers were up to date with progress and handed out brochures to all and sundry. Bookings began to come in.

We don't remember at which precise point John decided that 28 May 1994 would be the day in which the first family would be welcomed over the doorstep by the family helper – incurably optimistic, or as Kit sometimes said "unrealistic" about the rate of progress, he was determined to fill in as many weeks as possible in that opening year. In no time at all 19 families were booked in.

An advert was placed in the *Tenby Observer* for a family helper. In order to interview the applicants we came and stayed in Lower Albion for a week at the end of the Easter holidays. Kit showed each one around the still unfinished apartment above, and John and Jo Blackburn conducted more formal interviews. There was one obvious choice – Ruth Griffiths – who had all the qualities of humour and sensibility, alongside practical knowledge and skill, that we could have wished for.

All the hurdles were finally cleared and the home straight beckoned. Invitations to the opening were sent out and arrangements finalised. The finishing touches of artwork were chosen and hung in place. John Cahill, a local artist, generously donated a limited edition print of one of his distinctive paintings of Tenby harbour. At last all was ready.

CHAPTER 11

A Grand Opening

'Joy and Woe are woven fine,
Under every grief and pine
Runs a joy with silken twine.'
William Blake (1757–1827) – *Auguries of Innocence*, 1789

'HARRIET'S HOUSE' WAS finally completely adapted and furnished and, on Saturday, 21 May 1994 some 200 people assembled in Castle Square for the opening ceremony. We had managed to get the square clear of cars for perhaps the first time before or since. The only problem was that the suite of furniture for the living room had not arrived. Together with Angela and her husband John, with their sons David and Gethyn and Harriet's uncle Arthur and auntie Joan, we were sitting in a café overlooking the harbour for a well earned coffee, having prepared the house for viewing, when a white van arrived with the suite. We all leapt out of our seats, ran across the square, seized the furniture from the van and, throwing the packaging back into it, we carried the settee and chairs into the house. Before the opening Vera and Trevor Davies, who had bought 1 Laston House (part of the old bathhouse) from David, gave a lunch for some of the invited guests. It was intended that some of the food would be heated up in the kitchen of Harriet's House. In the midst of rising tension, however, Angela and Joan could not work out how to turn the oven on so the food was farmed out to various kitchens around the harbour. Apparently it was then smuggled red hot into Laston House amid whispers of "Don't tell Kit". Unfortunately, Vera had decorated the doorway of her house with welcoming balloons, and many people arriving into the square thought that they were also invited and the house was soon full to overflowing. Roger, who had worked on the property below No.1, was concerned about the weight on the floor, and so chose to forego the meal but his fears were unfounded, and there was no further drama for Vera to contend with that day.

As patron of the Trust, Bishop Dewi Bridges blessed and opened the house and, in doing so, paid tribute to Harriet saying that it was in honour of the memory of a very remarkable young girl. He added: "What better year than the Year of the Family to be opening Harriet's House? This fulfils Harriet's dream – a dream has become reality." Thanking him, John welcomed everybody and also thanked all those individuals, organizations and charitable trusts who had contributed in any way. Then, Dr Sandy Cavenagh spoke very movingly when he said in his speech as the Trust's president:

> You might think that Harriet Davis' life was the ultimate tragedy. She arrived comparatively late in life to John and Kit who, by a strange quirk of fate, knew more about the development of youth and handicapped children than any of us are likely to know. For a few months all went well and then the insidious signs of Leigh's Encephalopathy began. This is such a rare illness that a mere half dozen cases exist in the UK at any one time. It is due to a defect in an enzyme in the nervous system and the sufferer becomes weak and totally incapacitated. Weakness in swallowing necessitates tube feeding and poor breathing results in recurrent pneumonia, leading eventually to death.
>
> Until Harriet, the longest survival rate was to the age of seven.
>
> This was the appalling fate which befell Harriet and Kit and John. But the eventual results were not tragic at all. By some miracle, her intelligence, courage and humour were preserved to the last, and due to the superhuman efforts of her parents,

of the team at Neville Hall Hospital, Abergavenny, and her many helpers at home, she survived until the age of eleven. During this time her parents seldom had a night's sleep and they provided care beyond what the best-staffed hospital in the world could offer. The result was an inspiration to her family and friends and to all who came in touch with her.

And it did not end there. By their efforts in fund-raising John and Kit have sent £70,000 to the Research Trust for Metabolic Diseases in Children and £130,000 towards the Harriet Davis Seaside Holiday Trust, providing many families with similar problems with rest and recuperation in the specially equipped seaside holiday home.

I suspect we should judge the value of a life not only by its length, but by the amount of love it generates. In those terms Harriet was a centenarian. Her name will remain in perpetuity – or as least as long as Tenby stands – and her illness and life have made at least one not very Christian practitioner ponder anew the meaning of immortality.

Sandy did not, of course, mention his own role in Harriet's care which was magnificent and for which we will always be grateful. He never failed to call when asked; in fact he often popped in when passing on a Sunday afternoon, sometimes with granny and accompanying Great Dane in the car. He never made us feel that we were a nuisance and Harriet was always very pleased to see her uncle Sandy.

David Manby also spoke and, with a tear in his eye, admitted that he could not have achieved what we had done with the house. The pink ribbon, held by David and Gethyn, was ceremoniously cut by the bishop and the supporters were invited in to see what had been achieved.

Afterwards the Tenby Mothers' Union of St Mary's Church very kindly provided a buffet for all those who had come and this provided an opportunity to thank many friends. Anyone who has ever had dealings with the Mothers' Union know that their catering for such occasions is of a very high standard with delicious scones, welsh cakes and sandwiches in abundance. We cannot recall who arranged for the Mothers' Union to provide the tea, but still marvel at their generosity. Subsequently, we have spoken about the Trust to branches of the Union in the area and received great support from them.

After the excitement of the opening day, Harriet's House settled quietly to await the most important people – the families coming on holiday. They came from near and far: north-west Pembrokeshire, Breconshire, south Wales, the Midlands, with Surrey representing south-east England. We were pleased with the spread. Nineteen families, we felt, was an encouraging beginning. Some we already knew, others who returned again and again we came to know well. Ruth used to call to see each family during the week; remarks in the Visitors' Book made clear how much they welcomed her help and friendly manner.

Among the first was Gwyneth Humphries with her adoptive parents Joe and Shirley. Gwyneth, who suffered from spinabifida, had become Harriet's friend when they met during our brief early visits to the hydrotherapy pool in Brecon. When Harriet grew out of her first Turbo wheelchair, it was recycled to her. They used to enjoy meeting up and driving round the local play area together. Ben Gunnell came with George and Gwen, also adoptive parents. We came to know them very well and admired their dedication to Ben who was profoundly disabled. They continued to visit every year, helping also with fund-raising and some expert carpentry from George. Gwyneth and Ben are two of five children from the opening year who have since sadly died. After many years of holidaying with the Trust their lives are remembered with trees planted for them in the Star Meadow at the Wheelabout.

Malcolm and Margaret Melhuish, with their daughter Laura, came on holiday during that first August. The front door was open when they arrived and Malcolm ventured in. He looked at the living room and hurried back out to Margaret. "We've come to the wrong one," he said. "This is somebody's private house." We could not have been paid a finer compliment. Ruth, who had been putting the final touches to the 'special' bedroom, came hurrying out to reassure them that they had indeed found the right house. They also have become great friends and helpers, both to us personally and to Harriet's Trust with Malcolm, latterly, being able to serve as one of the Trustees of the charity. He has spent many hours in the houses decorating, carrying out repairs and gardening. Margaret often acts as a personal shopper for the Trust, making visits to large retail outlets such as IKEA for replacement items.

Ruth, now retired, still receives letters and cards from some of 'her' families. Sarah Griffiths, another adopted child, came in 1994 and continues to do so out of the main holiday season. She writes regularly to keep Ruth and us up to date with her life; as a young adult she is a keen supporter of all who are disabled and a scourge of politicians and authorities who are lax in their responsibilities to those like her. She's unafraid to speak out and take her place in society.

Back home we had to continue raising funds to pay David the final £10,000 of the purchase price and to build up a reserve for future expenses. We hoped that the modest letting charges would cover the running costs but realised that major repairs and replacements would have to be met from other monies. Having achieved what we set out to do there were no thoughts of providing anything further. We should have remembered the words of the Roman poet Horace, who obviously knew a thing or two. In one of his epistles from more than a thousand years ago he wrote:

Dimidium facti qui coepit habet, sapere aude.
To have begun is half the job; be bold and sensible.

Interlude
by Jo Blackburn

I first met Harriet and Kit very early in 1983 at the hydrotherapy pool at Ysgol Penmaes in Brecon when, as the newly appointed Development Officer for the Pre-School Playgroups' Association in Powys, I was getting to know the volunteers and families' groups that were part of the PPA organization in Powys. I was visiting the Brecon group in a hall in Llanfaes which had access to the pool. I vividly remember that first meeting – Harriet's auntie Joan was with them at the time, providing additional support for Kit when Harriet used the pool facilities. I was moved – Harriet was seemingly helpless and frail at that time and was in need of the round the clock care that Kit and John and others were providing. At the same time I also met John who, in his role as Community Development Officer, had responsibility for many of the Local Education Authority premises where many of the PPA groups met.

As I got to know Kit and John, I also got to know the large number of individuals who made up Harriet's support team. Granny Roberts (Kit's mother), auntie Joan and uncle Arthur, the Angelas, Rose and Alva, Liz and Gilly, a whole range of health care professionals, and the cats who were always in attendance, all contributed to the lively, but often anxious atmosphere in the home. My family's involvement also grew. Although Oliver and Edward were eight and four years older than Harriet, they soon became part of her circle of friends – where the boys outnumbered the girls. At Harriet's birthday parties, which conveniently coincided with Halloween and where pumpkin lanterns were always a feature, Jennifer Barnes was often the only other girl!

When Harriet was well enough and days out were possible, Kit, John and Harriet often visited us, and outings and picnics were arranged. On one visit to the National Museum of Wales in Cardiff during half-term, Harriet was thrilled as huge beasts loomed and snarled in murky corners – while many older children ran whimpering to the exit, seeking consolation in the brightly lit entrance hall and the enticing gift shop. Harriet was always delighted to see our goats and their kids and they, in turn, welcomed her attention and returned her affection as goats do, with nibbles and gentle nudges.

In those far off days, the Research Trust for Metabolic Diseases in Children (RTMDC) was the charity we all helped to raise funds for. I well remember a carol singing expedition around our neighbours one Christmas, which raised a few pounds for the Trust, but proved that the Blackburn family was no match for the Von Trapps. On another occasion, Graham and I, with John's brother Paul and his wife Tina, represented the Brecon branch of RTMDC at a meeting with Members of Parliament at the House of Commons, to lobby for more funds for research into metabolic diseases in children.

More successful was the Fun Run, raising money for H's electric wheelchair, which we all took part in. Organized by Ivan Boreham we ran, jogged or just hobbled around the lanes of Llangynidr. My nephew, Daniel, joined us for the occasion and Sarah, our younger daughter, famously took a short cut and arrived at the finish well ahead of anyone else.

When Harriet died in 1992 all those who had been involved with previous fund-raising efforts rallied behind John and Kit and wholeheartedly supported their plan to honour Harriet's memory with the Seaside Holiday Trust. Fund-raising took on a new dimension and, once again, a range of events and initiatives drew in family, friends and neighbours for a cause that was so dear to our hearts. With the opening of Harriet's House on that famous day, when we all stood outside in bright sunshine and listened to the speeches, we were all aware that Harriet was the inspiration and Kit and John were the driving force that had made such a huge undertaking possible.

CHAPTER 12

Fingers Crossed

'In for a penny, in for a pound'
Seventeenth-century proverb

ALMOST AS SOON as Harriet's House on the harbour began to be used, we were overwhelmed with the demand for the following year from families desperate for a place to stay which would meet their needs. We found that, in commercial terms, we had uncovered a previously untapped 'market' of families with disabled children wanting holiday accommodation that was properly adapted and equipped for them – a demand which far outstripped the modest facility we had provided.

It was after the National Lottery began that we seriously considered buying and adapting a second house for the Trust. Initially we had wanted the responsibility of only the one house, but the prospect of securing a large grant to buy another property was very enticing. With two houses we confidently expected to satisfy the demand for holidays from our rapidly growing base of families. In 1996 we were one of the first applicants to the National Lottery Charities Board in their third round of awards, as disability, alongside health and care, was one of its programme areas. John sent for application forms from the Charities Board in Wales – lengthy and detailed, these presented his skills with another challenge.

The expected application pack arrived; a fifty-page booklet of instruction and explanation designed to help with filling in the actual twenty-page application form consisting of some sixteen multi-part questions. Full details had to be given about the project finances: how much we were asking for, when we intended to start, and how the rest of the money was to be raised. Information about the number of voluntary helpers, paid staff, copies of our accounts and Trust deed, together with a business plan were needed. An additional building or refurbishment form also had to be completed. John went out, bought a plentiful supply of cigarettes and peppermints to draw upon in stressful moments, and set about the task.

Discussion with the other Trustees and a close look at the then current property market in Tenby led to a total estimated project cost of a little under £149,000; of this we decided to ask the lottery for £110,500 to buy a suitable property. The Trust already had access to £26,000 towards the outstanding £39,000. We all felt confident in our ability to raise the remainder within the required time limit. Having cut our teeth on Harriet's House, the task ahead was more exciting than daunting. A little knowledge can indeed lead to overconfidence.

Once again, forms completed and posted, we had metaphorically cast our bread upon the waters and waited to see if we would find any return. A letter of acknowledgement of our application arrived at the end of July 1996. Hard upon its heels came the first problem lying in wait for us on what we had naively expected to be a rather smooth path to success.

An assessor from the Welsh board of the lottery went through our forms in meticulous detail. His chief query concerned the question of trustees. "Why", he wanted to know, "is there no user-family represented amongst your trustees?" Lengthy telephone conversations followed, as John tried to explain that this situation was not of our choosing. In October 1992 we had been clearly told by the Charity Commission that the relevant charity law stated that no trustee of a charity could also be a beneficiary. In our case this meant that the family of such a trustee would be unable to use the Trust property for a holiday – not something guaranteed to attract volunteers. Kit also privately voiced the opinion that many parents of disabled children are fully stretched, emotionally and physically, and would find it difficult to take on extra responsibilities.

The assessor, unconvinced, gave us the feeling that this ruling would count against us when decisions about grant allocations were made. Were we to fall at this first unexpected hurdle? John's years of experience in dealing with administrative problems in the community now gave him an advantage. Letters were passed between the Trust, the Charity Commission, the Association of Voluntary Organizations in Powys, and the Lottery Charities Welsh board. Telephone calls were made and received: John's cigarette and peppermint consumption climbed. A letter then, dated 31 October 1996, from the Charity Commission stated:

> ... There is nothing to stop parents of disabled children acting as charity trustees now but they will have to observe the rule that they must not take any material benefit for themselves or their children and they will have to observe the provisions of clause 14(b) of the governing instrument. We would, if a case is made out, be willing to establish the necessary scheme to permit parents to act as charity trustee and take benefits subject to there being an agreed regime of declaration of interests...

The letter also stated that this would entail making a case 'to demonstrate that the charity was unable to function effectively unless user trustees were appointed and that its work would thus be unduly hampered...' For us the nub of the letter and of most importance, was contained in the concluding words:

> This [the case] could be shown if the experience of the charity was that not only the NLCB (National Lottery Charities Board) but other grant-givers and institutional supporters (such as local authorities) had failed or were reluctant to lend support to this body without such trustees...

The assessor pronounced himself satisfied, we held a muted celebration at successfully clearing this hurdle, but knew that this in itself was no guarantee to achieving a grant.

At last, on 11 December 1996 came a letter with the all-important opening words: 'I am pleased to inform you that the National Lottery Charities Board has agreed...' It had been a long six months but we had been awarded the £110,500 that we had asked for. Now we could properly celebrate before getting down to all the practicalities involved. The excitement bubbled up afresh as we made the first trip to view properties that we thought might be suitable for adaptation. At the same time we continued to apply for grants towards the furnishing and equipment that we would need. We travelled to London for a day to visit the NADEX (National Association for Disability Exhibition) show to look at new products and came home with bags full of brochures and minds full of information to be sorted. Fund-raising events couldn't be forgotten either. Harriet's House needed time and attention to maintain a good standard as well as dealing with booking families in for their holidays. Life was busy, but satisfying and interesting.

We looked at many houses in Tenby and around the area, becoming quite expert in quickly deciding what would work for our purposes and what would not. We particularly remember visits to a penthouse apartment (what were we thinking of?), an old convent building (far too big), and a small hotel (full of bri-nylon bedding, dust and with what can only be described as an eccentric approach to fire escape provision). Roger Toms came with us on occasions and bounced on floors and inspected attics before giving us his professional opinion as to the feasibility of adapting the places for the use intended. "If you want this one you're on your own. I'm not touching it," he stated more than once with a hiss of indrawn breath between his front teeth that only fully fledged builders have the ability to master. In a nearby village, at another viewing, the bathroom boasted a blue steel bath; Kit disgracefully began to giggle as Roger pointed it out and raised his eyebrows murmuring "David's bath?" as he did so. Making a smart exit from the house, Kit carefully closed the back door behind her. The owner of the house was standing outside talking to John. It was a cold, blustery day and the man was in his shirt sleeves – no coat. "You haven't shut the door?" he called anxiously. "Yes" said Kit eager to make a good impression after the giggling episode. "It's a Yale lock and I haven't got a key on me," he almost wailed. We left him seeking sanctuary at a nearby friend's house and made a hasty escape.

At last we found an ideal property – David Manby came with us to the estate agent. To our surprise he produced his chequebook and made a respectable cash offer for a quick sale. Equally surprising to us, the offer was rejected and then we were told that the property was no longer on the market. We began to feel a little anxious. Would we manage after all to find the right property and complete our project in the allotted time?

Ruth Griffiths and Kit viewed two houses together. One, a guest house, was full of cheap ornaments covering every available flat surface, with walls equally adorned. Safely outside again, the mounting hysteria brought on by the sheer volume of ornaments exploded into laughter. We managed at last to make a shortlist of three possibilities which all the Trustees came down to view on one day. Ruth came too, but refused to come in again to the ornamented guest house as she was afraid that she and Kit might not be able to contain themselves this time.

Everyone, at last, agreed that Giltar View in Southcliffe Street, close to the large Rectory Car Park, was the one. Roger was happy with our choice; an offer of £90,000 was accepted. The house is a typical late Victorian terraced town house of three storeys; from the first floor there is a view over the car park to the sea and South Beach, no garden but an enclosed yard at the back. Later we discovered that the house was the family home of Andrew Muskett, who later designed the Wheelabout for the Trust, and who, after leaving private practice, became one of our Trustees. It was interesting to learn from an old guide of Tenby town from the 1930s that the house had been used for bed and breakfast accommodation, something that the Muskett family had continued. So the tradition that the house would be used for holidaymakers would be maintained.

The surveyor who came to inspect the house looked up at the roof as he got out of his car. He immediately got back in and moved his vehicle to the opposite side of the road. "Roof needs replacing," he said briskly. Roger and his team set about gutting and remodelling the interior whilst the new roof was put on. There was also the need to install a lift to carry a wheelchair to the first floor where the 'special' bedroom and bathroom were to be situated. Once again Roger's team of men worked hard and enthusiastically. He was always ready to discuss and listen to their solutions to achieve the best result. During early summer we took our goddaughter, Sally, for her Tenby beach holiday. On one of the fine days that week, we were sitting enjoyably on South Beach watching her play in the sand when a 'runner' arrived from Southcliffe Street. "You're to come at once. You're needed at the house," was the breathless message. Fearing some awful accident, we left Sally and her mother enjoying the sands, and hastened up the steep ramp from the beach and across the car park to the house. Out of breath and expecting at least blood on the floor, if not worse, we were met by Michael, the carpenter. "You've got the kitchen and dining rooms the wrong way round," he said. "The kitchen should be at the very back – it will only need the windows replaced with suitable ones and it will be much better." Originally, the very back room had been used as a private family room when the house was a bed and breakfast establishment. For those of us without the knowledge of what is possible in the way of building works, it seemed that moving the position of a kitchen was a daunting task. Roger and his team made light work of it and it did not add much to the end cost of our project. After we had forgiven him for giving us such a heart-stopping race up from the beach, we agreed that Michael, the carpenter, was quite

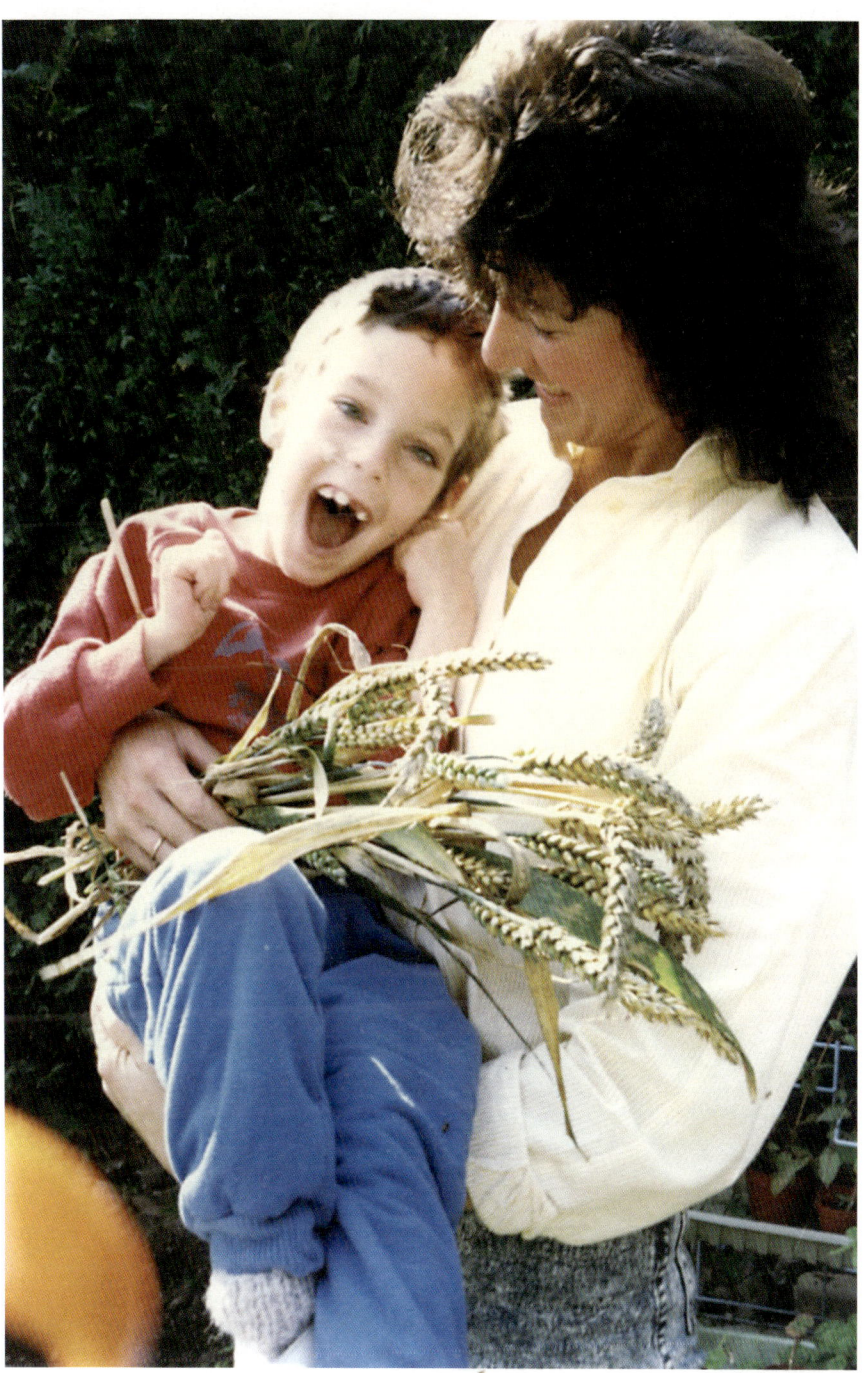

Gilly and Harriet at harvest time.

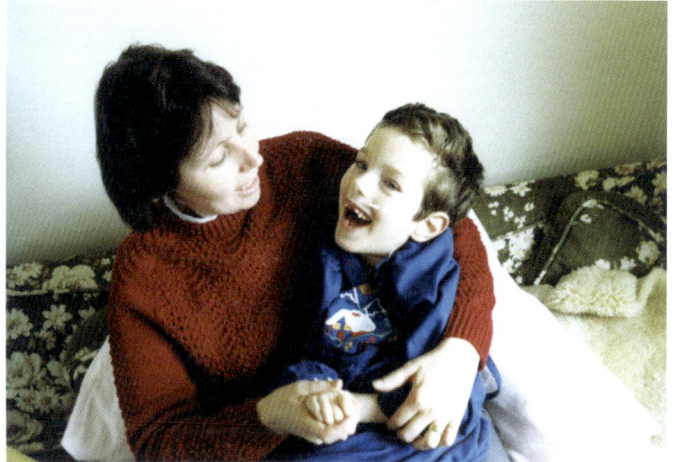

'Auntie' Rose Hopkins and Harriet enjoying being together.

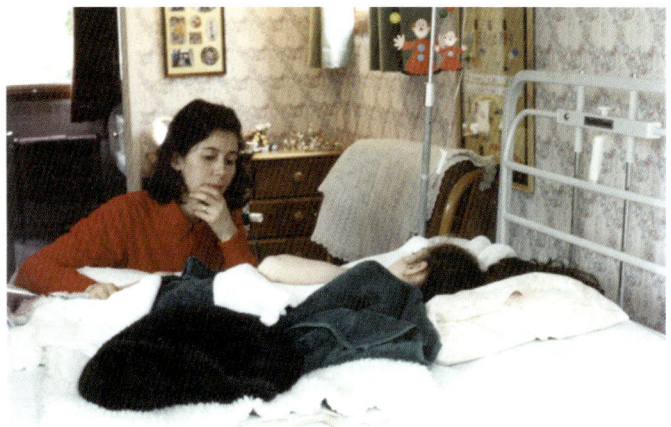

Alva, Harriet and black cat at the end of a long and difficult night shift.

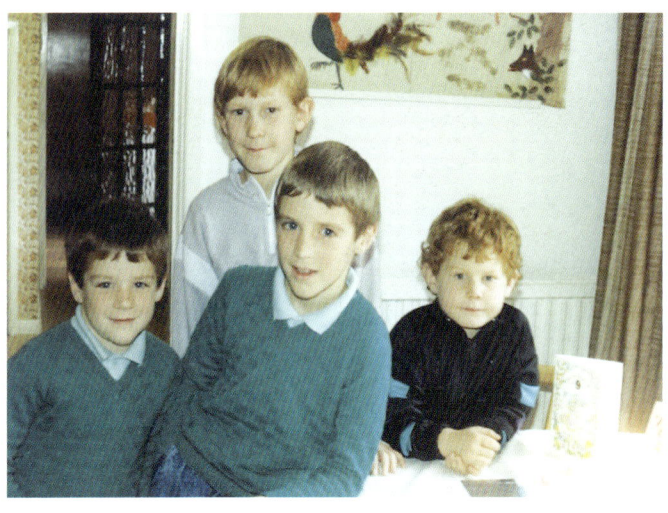

Harriet's 'best boys' 1989. L–R: Gareth and Rhydian Roberts at the back, Gethyn and David McFall at the front.

Driving lesson in new Turbo with Jan Boreham.

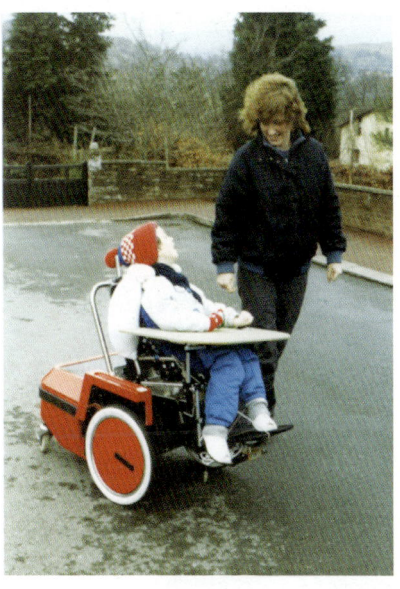

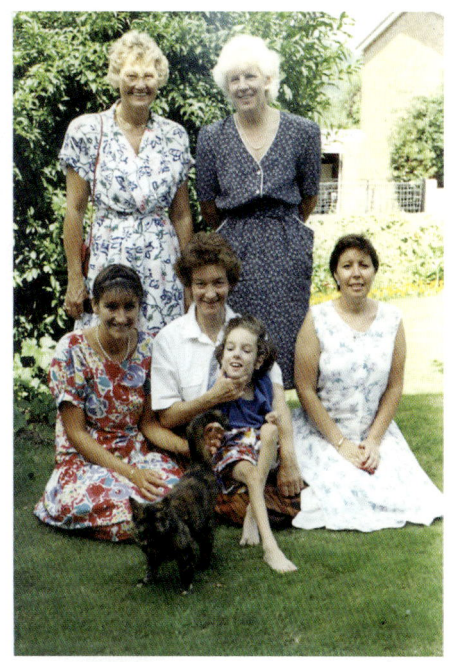

Hospital friends. L–R standing: Sisters Rosemary Williams and Joan Hardman; kneeling: Alison Ward, nursery nurse, Kit and Harriet, staff nurse Rose Hopkins.

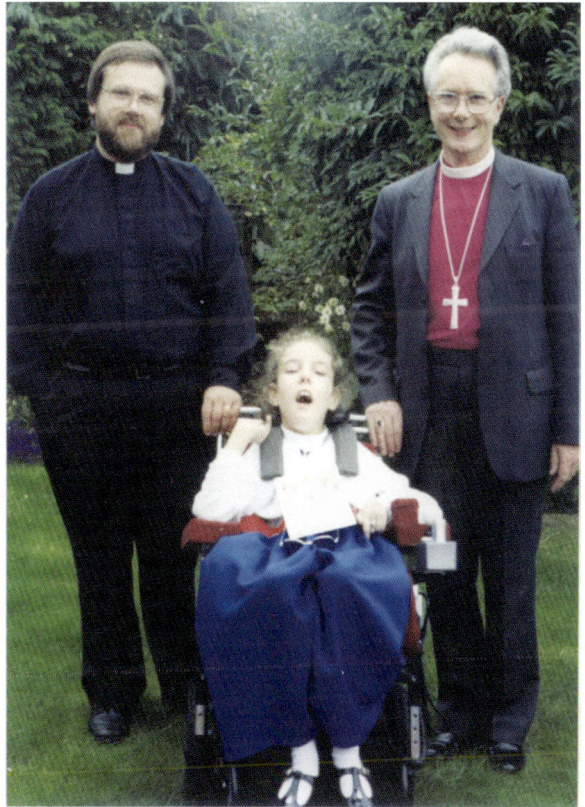

Confirmation Day, 17th December 1991, with Bishop Dewi Bridges and Rev. Kelvin Richards.

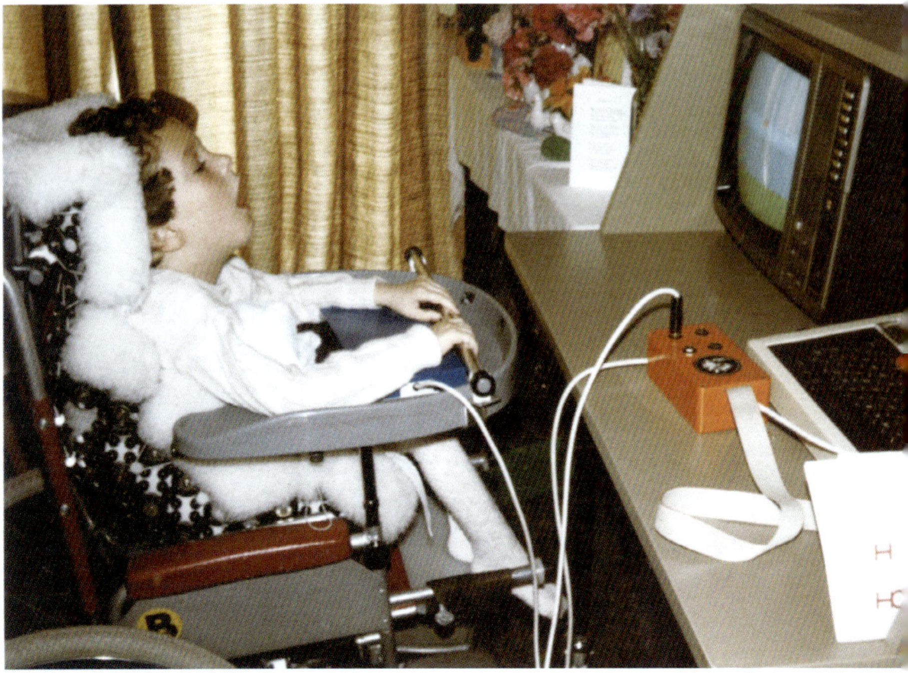

Early days on the computer.

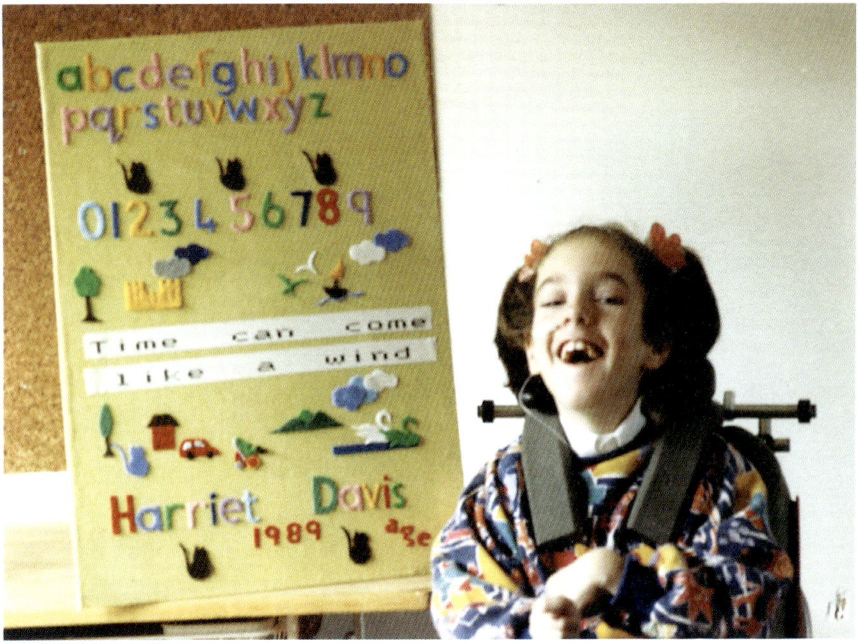

The finished sampler ready for framing.

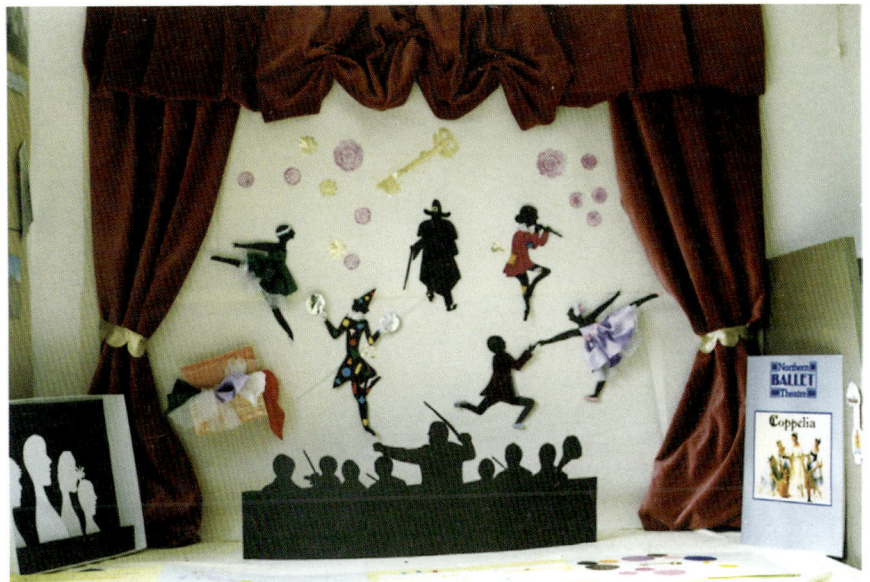

Coppelia table prepared before visit to the ballet.

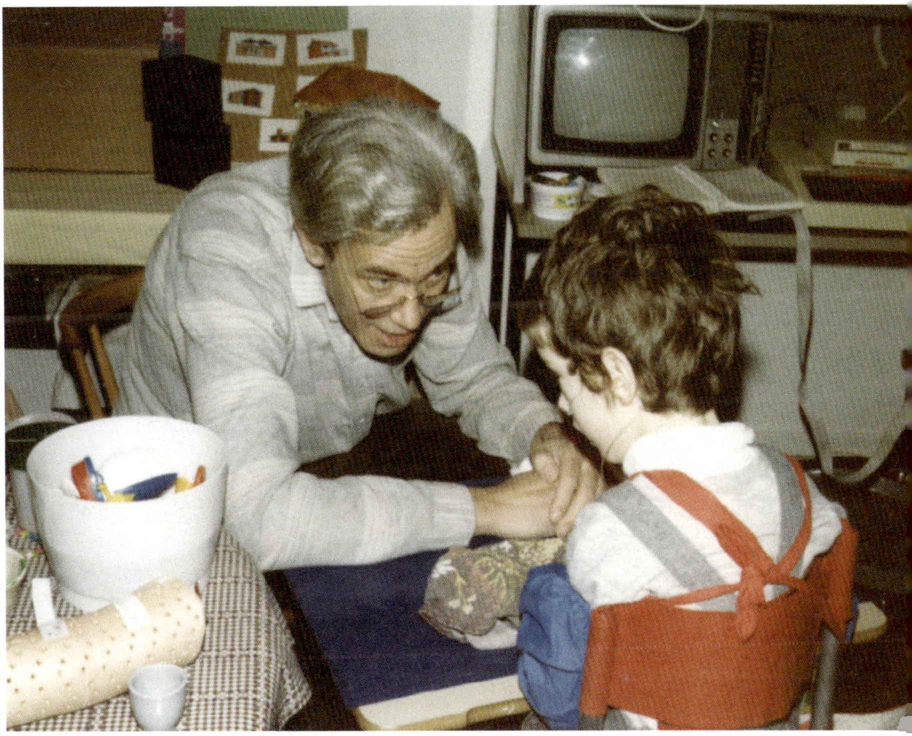

Chatting to Daddy.

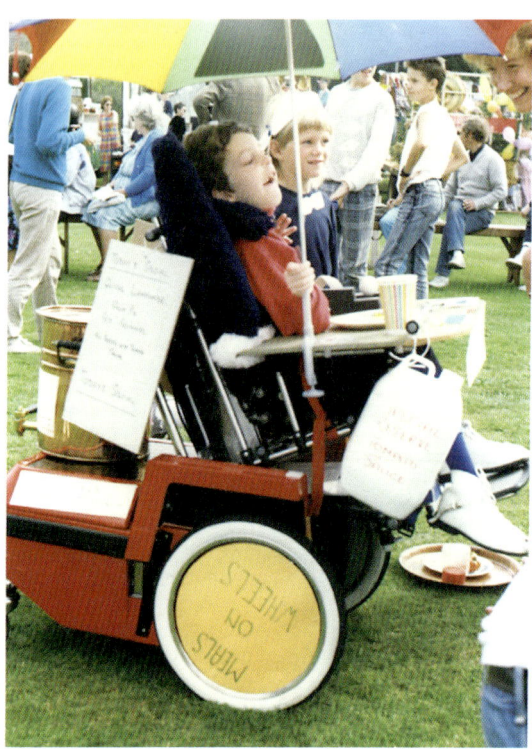

Llangynidr Gala 'meals on wheels' with Jennifer Barnes as the nippy waitress.

A walk with Gilly near the Brecon Beacons' Mountain Centre.

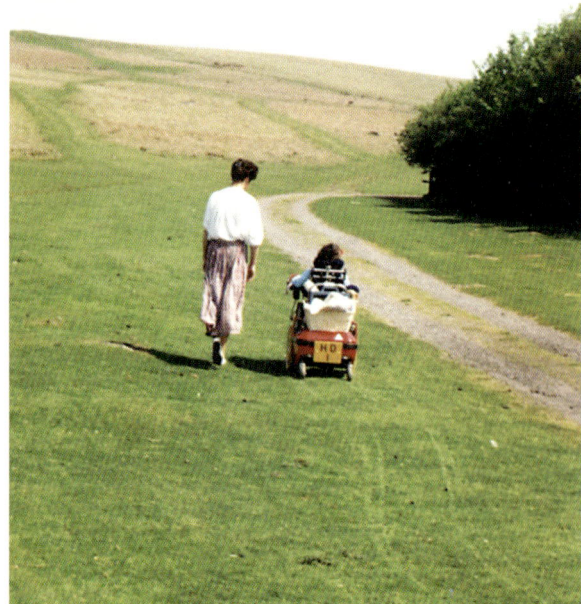

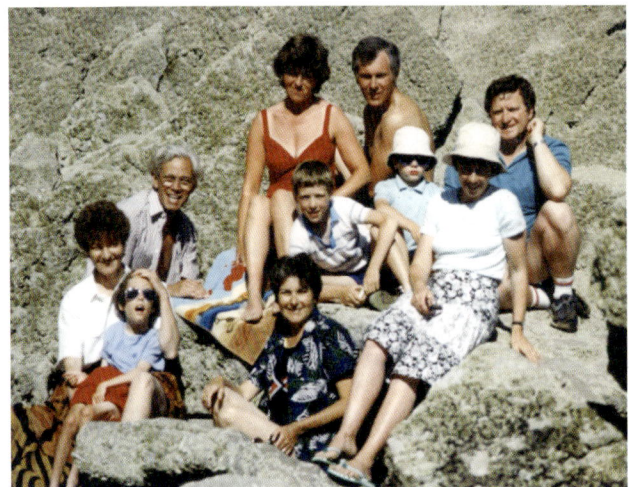

On the beach at Tenby in 1989. L–R cousins Christine and Alan with the Davis family and Auntie Joan and the McFall family.

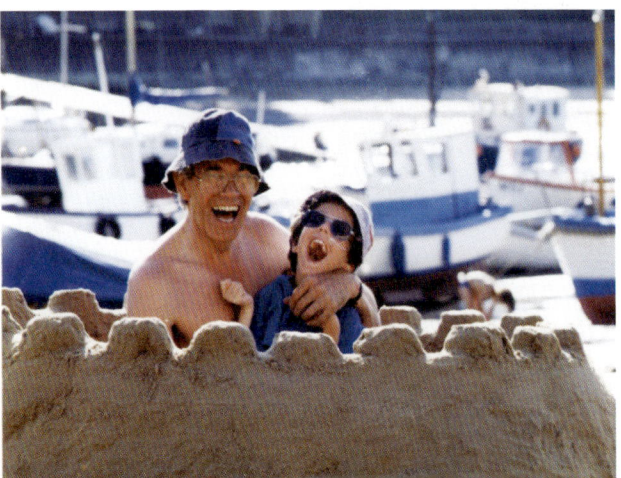

John and Harriet in the sandcastle on Tenby harbour.

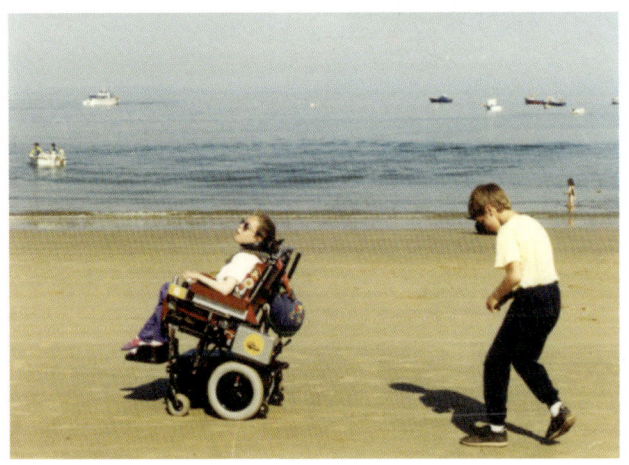

Driving on North Beach, Tenby with David in pursuit.

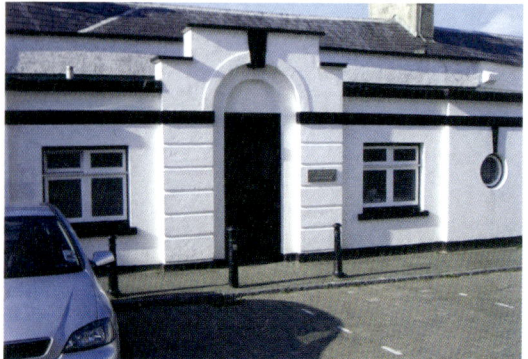

Harriet's House, overlooking Tenby harbour, opened in 1994.

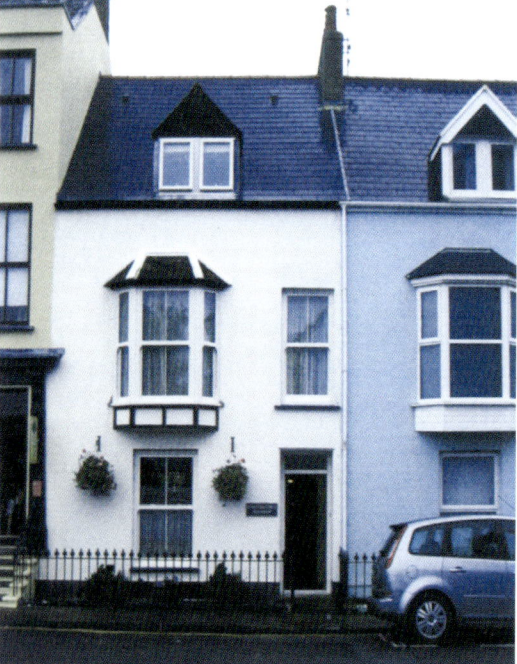

Giltar View, Southcliffe Street, Tenby, opened in 1998.

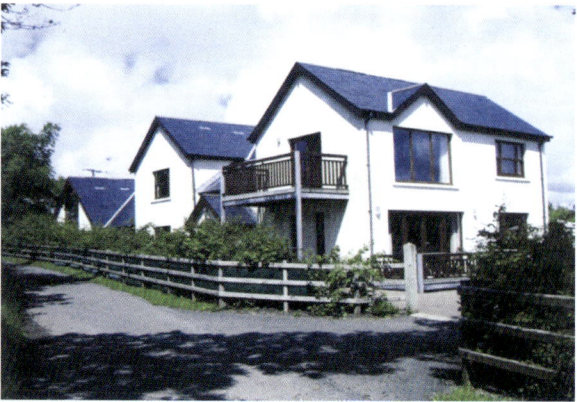

The Wheelabout, Strawberry Lane, Penally, opened in 2002.

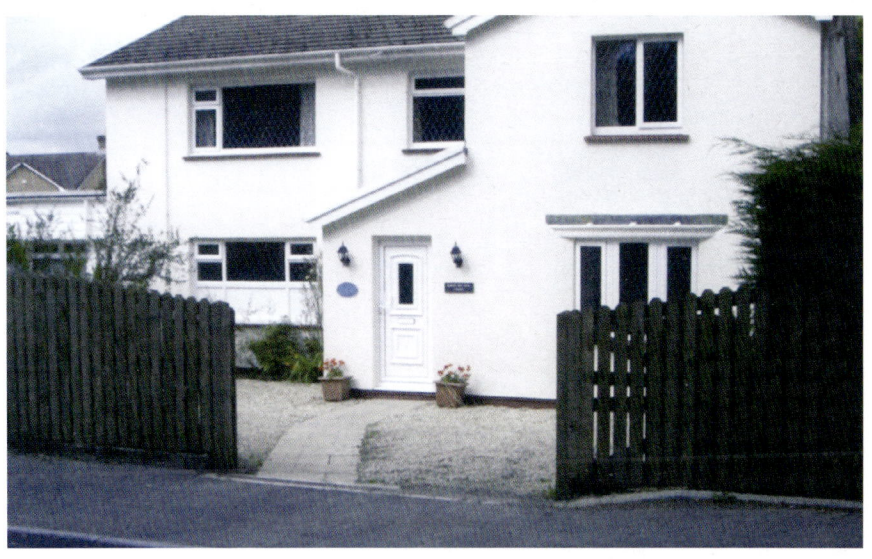

Caerwen, Jesse Road, Narberth, opened in 2008.

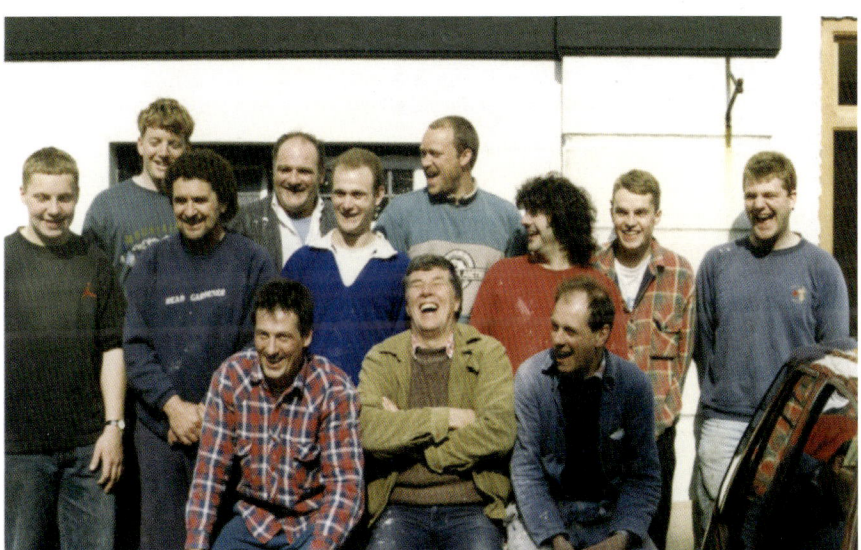

Enjoying a break from the building works at Harriet's House in 1993. Roger Toms (centre) with his team.

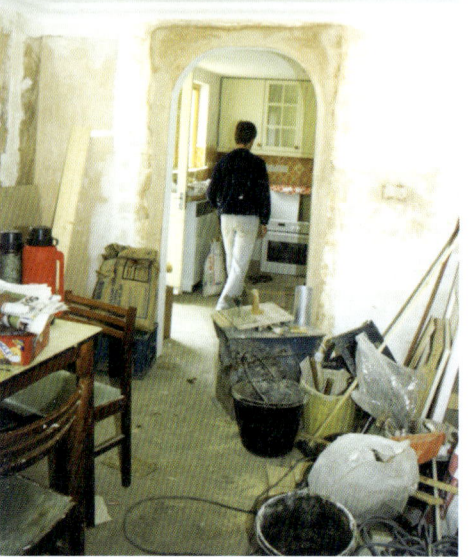

Renovations at Giltar View: new kitchen and dining room.

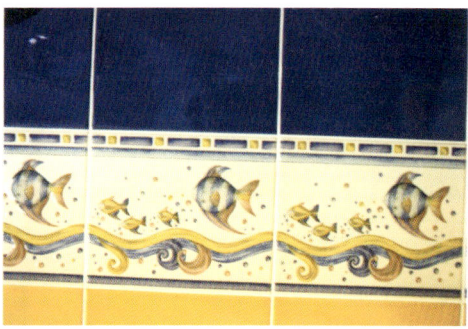

Fishy frieze from Turkey, Giltar View bathroom.

The Wheelabout's construction. John, no words needed!

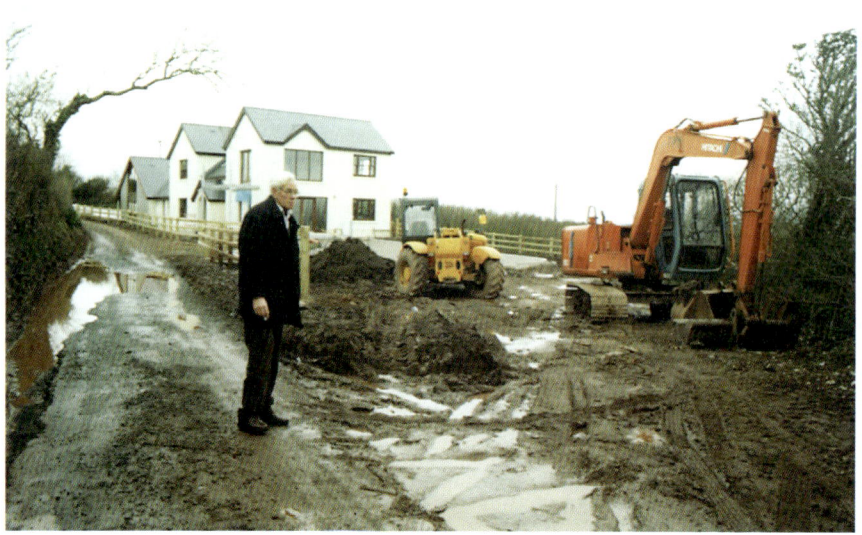

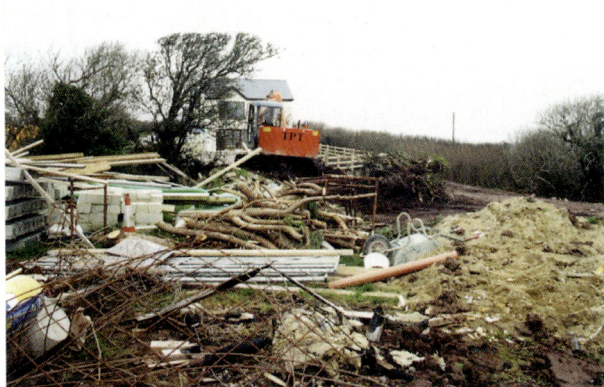

"Don't make a mess of the field." A failed instruction.

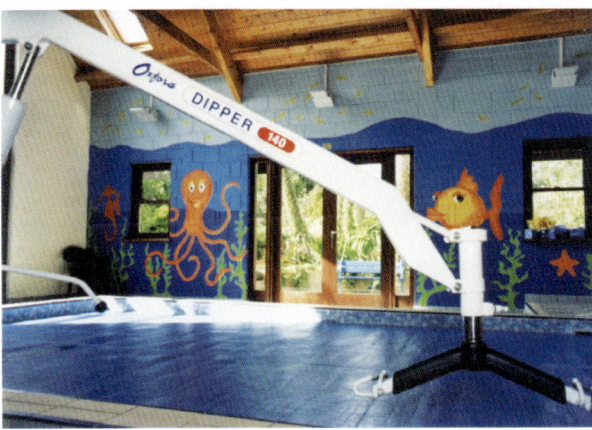

The Wheelabout swimming pool and mural.

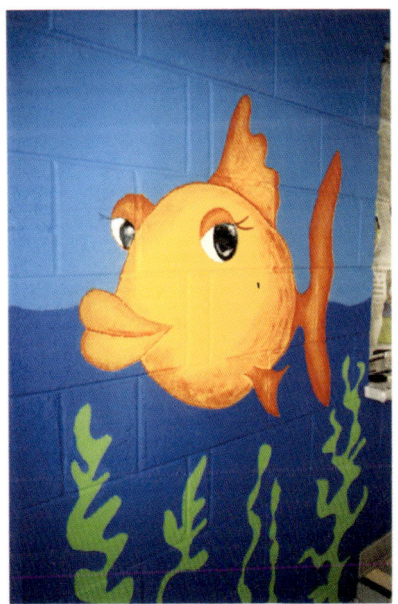

Close-up of 'Seductive Sid'.

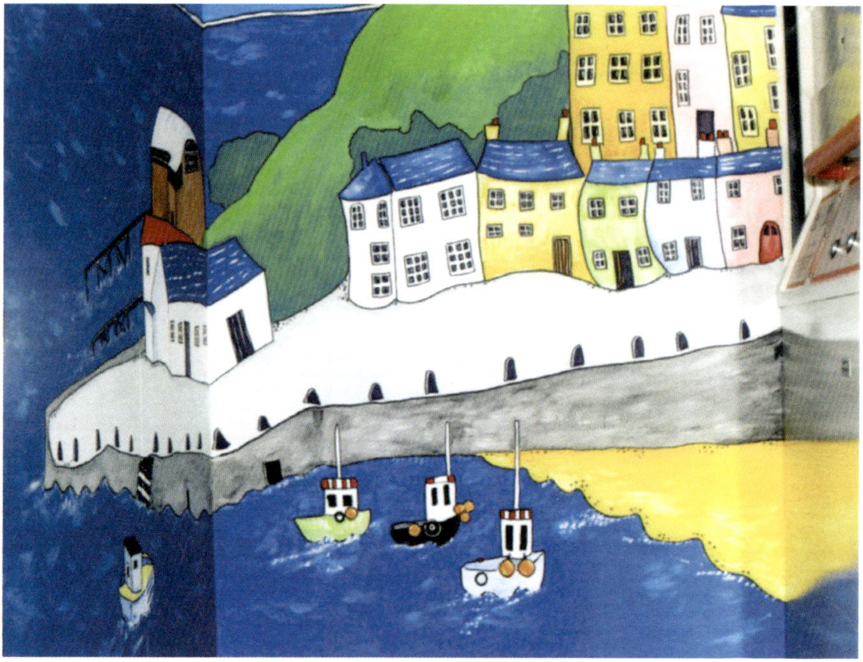

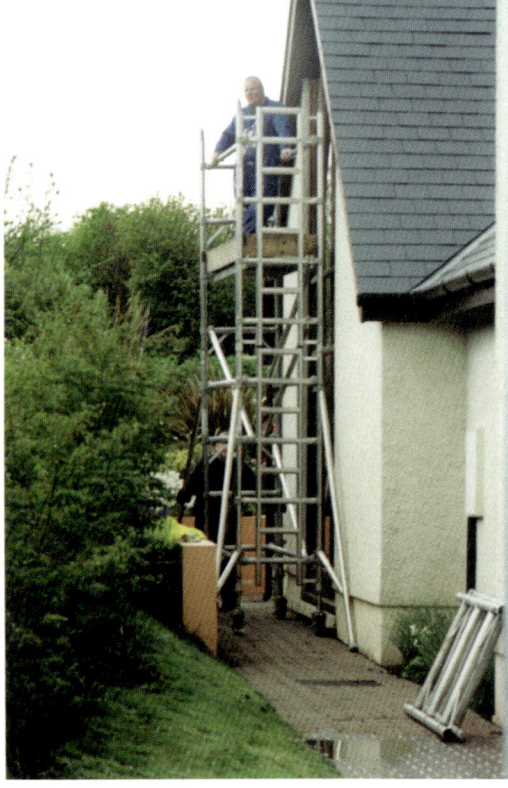

Jo Thomas's decoration of the Wheelabout lift shaft.

Activity week – Malcolm and the scaffolding tower.

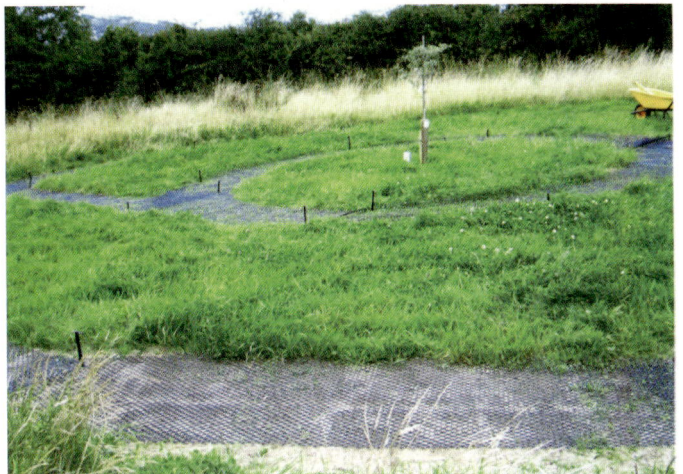

Wheelchair friendly paths under construction.

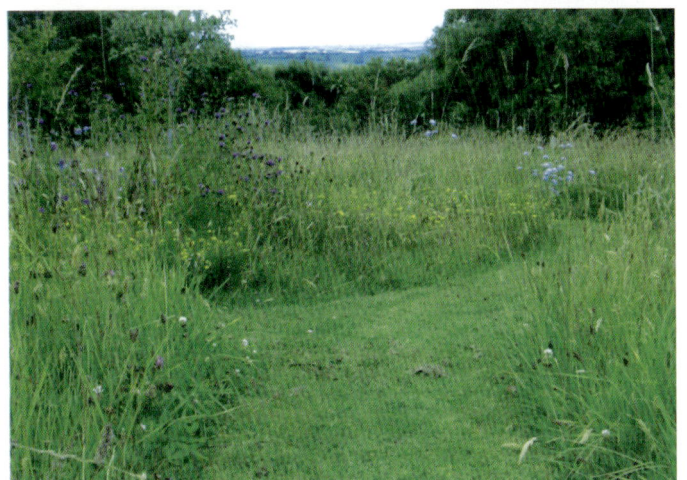

Meadow paths, 2010.

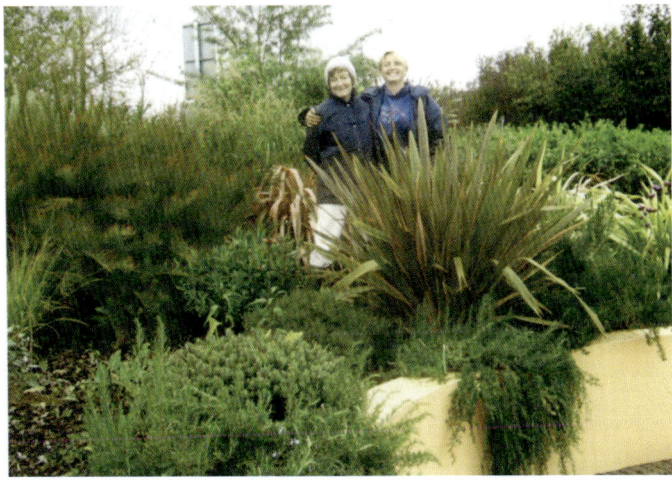

The 'Ancient Free Gardener' and Jenny Axon, her young assistant.

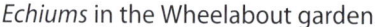
Echiums in the Wheelabout garden.

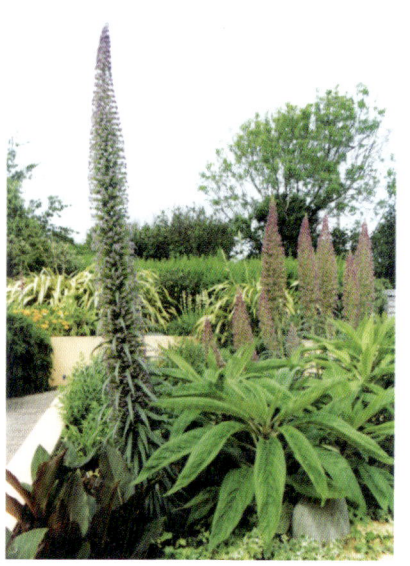

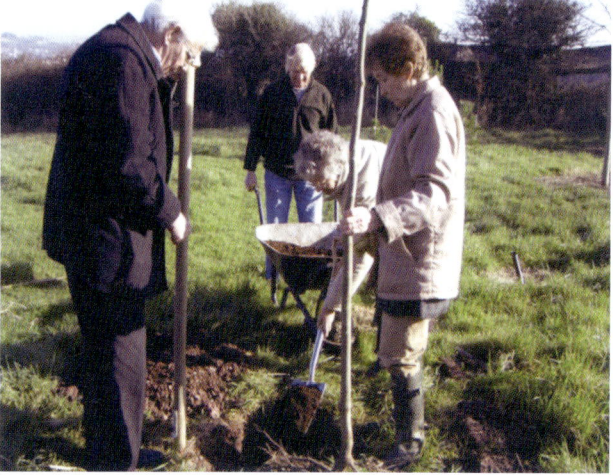
Planting a commemorative tree.

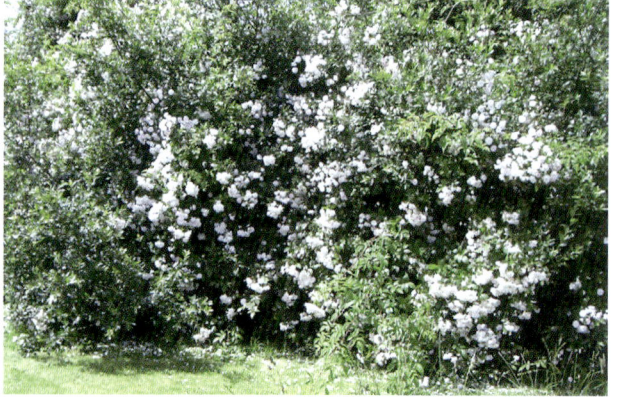
Himalayan Musk Rose in the meadow, June 2011.

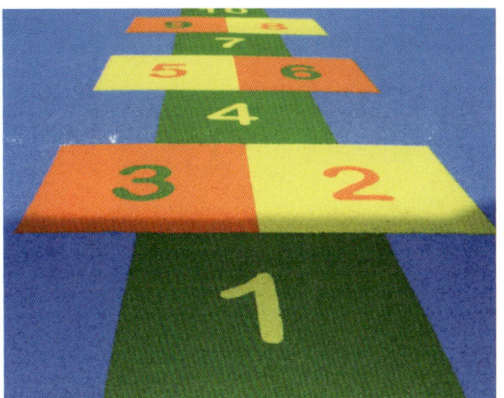

Hop Scotch at Caerwen.

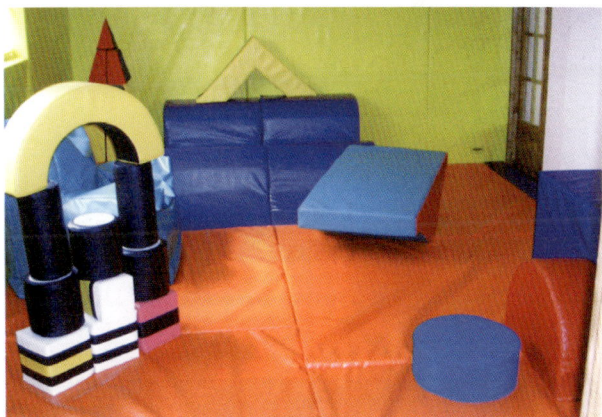

The soft playroom at Caerwen.

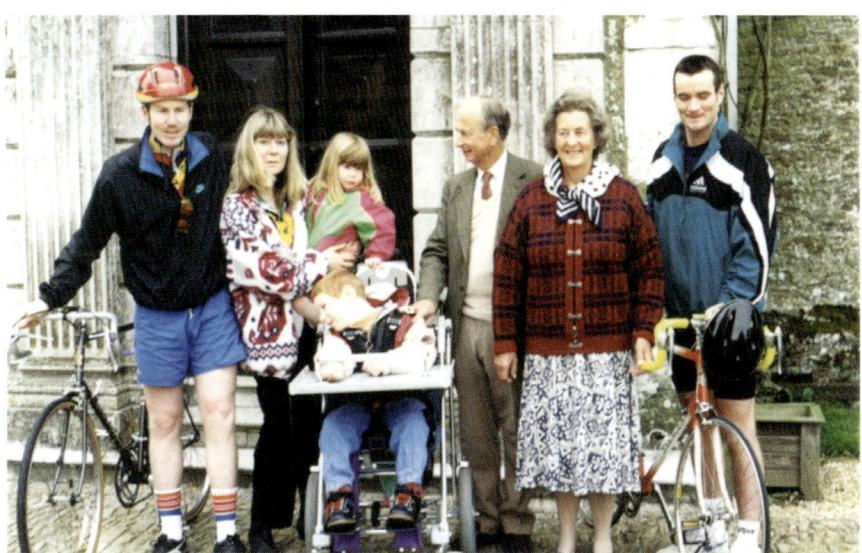

Bicycle ride from Loseley Park, Guildford to Tenby. Major and Mrs James More-Molyneux with the Kaffenberger family and Mark Sieven.

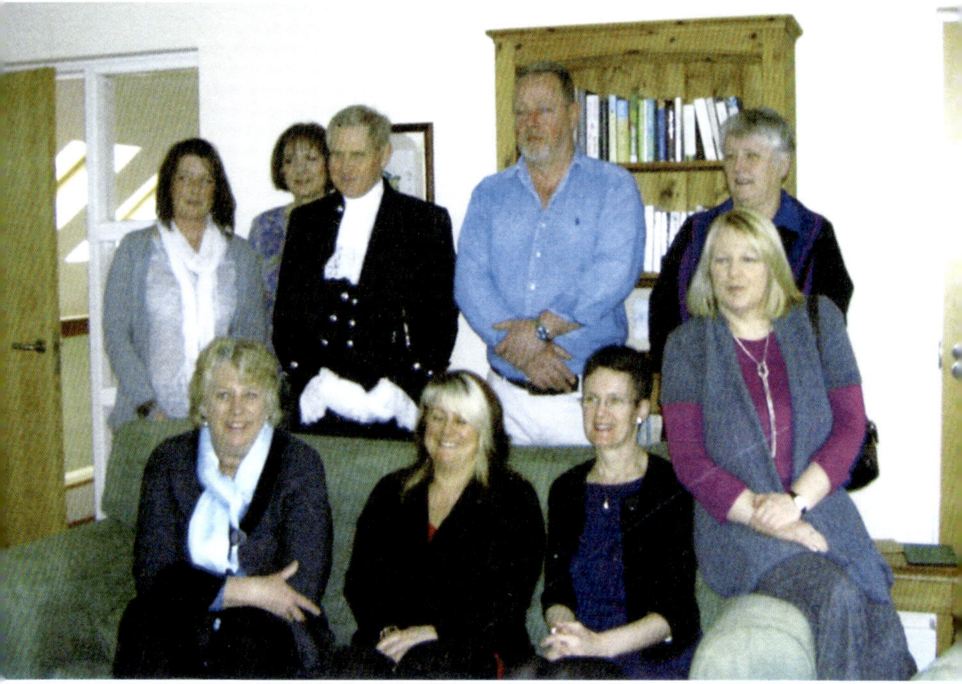

Presentation of the High Sheriff's Award to the Trust in 2010. Mr David Pryse Lloyd with the Trust's staff.

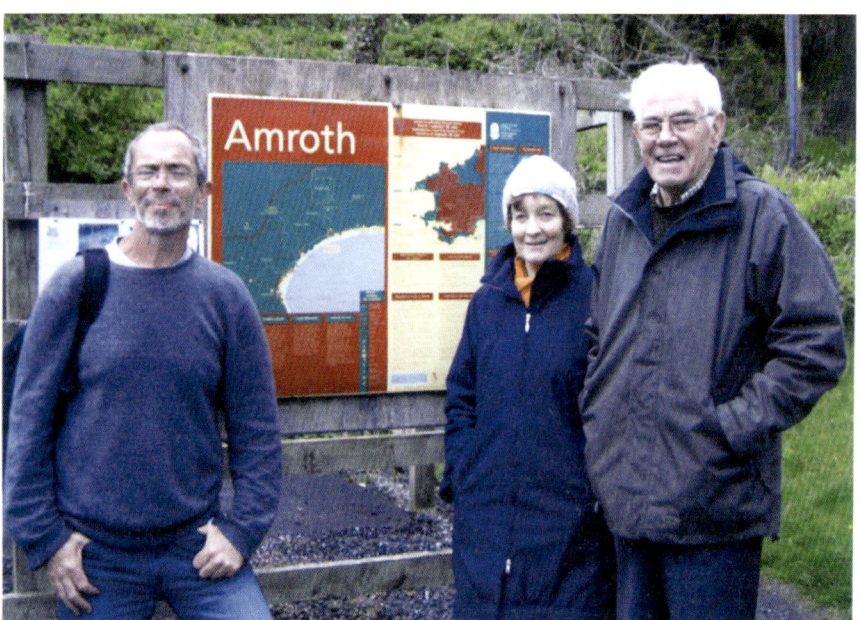

James Masterman at the end of his week's walk along the Pembrokeshire Coastal Path in 2010.

right. The resiting of the kitchen gave a much better 'flow' to the house.

The lift was another major part of the building works. The measurements involved were critical and the technical details beyond us. We were only too relieved to let Roger do the worrying – which he undoubtedly did – knowing that the lift was of fundamental importance to the success of the project. Once again good team management between builder, steel fabricator, and lift manufacturer produced the goods. The lift fitted perfectly and worked. All was well, once again.

Kit chose bathroom and kitchen tiles, wallpaper, paint colours and had a thoroughly enjoyable time. The 'special' bedroom and adjoining bathroom were given a blue and yellow seaside theme. Vivid yellow walls in the bedroom, with a wide fishy border, was echoed by the blue and yellow bathroom tiles with a wide border tile of colourful embossed fish. These tiles were manufactured in Turkey: the plain colours arrived promptly, but the border tiles were obviously being transported on foot and failed to materialize until after the first families had used the house. The plumber's young worker (not used before or since) had indulged a ten-year-old schoolboy's sense of humour by writing what Kit deemed 'inappropriate words' on the wall space where the border tiles were to go. The young man was summoned to meet her at 8 a.m. on the morning following her inspection of the offending graffiti. He arrived and when taken to task was foolish enough to smirk at his scolding. Kit had spent too many years teaching recalcitrant boys to be fazed by this. Pithily dealing with both his sins of commission and omission (the radiator in the hall was leaking onto the newly-laid carpet), she dispatched him to the bathroom with a paintbrush and tin of magnolia emulsion paint to obliterate the words. Some time later, no longer smiling, the young man was sent back to report to his employer. As we were parking in the Rectory Car Park we looked across to the curtainless front window of the 'special' bedroom where the painter was busily working. The bright yellow of the walls shone like a beacon across the car park. Kit went up to see it at close quarters. "I think I've made a mistake, Dickie," she said to the decorator. "It's awfully bright." "Too late," said Dickie. "I'm not redoing it." Then, more kindly, he added, "It won't look so bad when the furniture and carpet and curtains are in."

We went to Cardiff and spent several hours in one of those retail shops that offer rolls of discontinued patterns, or slight seconds of furnishing materials. We rummaged, compared, asked for advice and deliberated. The pages of window measurements were consulted by the staff – lengthy calculations were made. Eventually we emerged from the shop with a copy of the order to make all the curtains for Giltar View except one pair – for the breakfast room – for which Kit had not found a suitable material. We felt very pleased with the cost savings involved and hoped that we would be as pleased with the finished product. A colourful blue and yellow pattern was the choice for the large south-facing 'special' bedroom. It would either help tone down the yellow walls or make them seem even brighter. We would have to wait and see.

Back in Tenby painting and decorating and carpet-laying continued. Norman's son, Adam, was given the job of repainting the black railings at the front of the house. Adam, in his late teens, always looked as if he had partied hard the night before, but would follow instruction if given clearly and patiently. The holiday season had started and a steady procession of people was heading along the pavement outside the house. John was concerned lest someone, brushing against the railings, would get black paint on their clothing. He took a piece of cardboard outside and gave it to Adam. "Put 'Wet Paint' on that Adam please," he said. Adam looked at John. Obviously thinking the old man had lost his senses Adam obligingly drew a brushful of gleaming, black, wet paint across the piece of card and handed it back to John, without saying a word. Equally wordlessly John took it and retreated back into the house to regroup, whilst the rest of the workforce howled with laughter.

July came and the work neared completion. This time John

had reined in his optimism about the number of families who could be accommodated in this first year of opening. Eight weeks had been allocated and Jayne Conbeer was engaged to look after the running of the house. She was young, lived nearby and, as a trained nursery nurse, had some experience with small children and disability. We felt that once again we had been lucky to find someone with a warm, caring personality who would be an asset to the Trust in our new venture. The first family was booked in for mid August.

Fred arrived from Abergavenny with two helpers and a van-load of furniture which we had purchased from his furnishing shop. It was a hot day and, despite our best efforts, time was beginning to be critical. On that same day there were in the house: the plumber, the builder, David and Gethyn McFall, their parents, John and Angela, Jo and Graham Blackburn, Mike and Anne Chamberlain, who had never failed to give us help from the time that Mike had driven us and Harriet to Great Ormond Street some sixteen years previously and, of course, ourselves. At least fourteen bodies spread throughout the house, all busy unwrapping goods, carrying furniture, putting finishing touches to paint, tightening screws and so on. Barely controlled chaos might best describe the atmosphere. Fred, tall in stature and rotund in frame, wedged himself in the lift with a large cupboard destined for the 'special' bedroom. Everyone in the house breathed in and held his or her breath as Fred sucked in his stomach. Gethyn, David and Fred's helpers (who stayed known only as Fred's helpers) waited for the lift to ascend and helped ease Fred and the cupboard out and into the bedroom. Everyone breathed out, in relief. We decided Mike Chamberlain, with his much slighter build, would travel up and down in the lift and Fred could stick to the stairs. The large pine dining table was placed into position and immediately all the chairs were occupied by 'workers', talking and drinking tea or lemonade. There is nothing better than a good, big, kitchen or dining table to foster conversation and idleness.

Fortunately we had already delayed the formal official

opening ceremony until the first week in October. Originally scheduled for late July, we had reluctantly realised that building work and time were not going to be on our side. We were disappointed that we would not have those all-important settling down days before the first family arrived on 16 August. But it was not to be. On the final Friday, Norman was busy laying the last of the paving slabs in the back yard where the walls had been newly-painted in a Mediterranean terracotta colour. As we left the house, Roger put the finishing touch to the small, shallow concrete ramp to the front door. "It'll be dry by tomorrow afternoon," he promised. It was 15 August – we had cut it very fine indeed.

The remarks in the Visitors' Book were reassuringly complementary and the rest of the summer passed without incident. On 4 October we gathered again for the official opening.

Unlike our celebration for the opening of Harriet's House in 1994, the gathering at Giltar View was altogether smaller and more intimate. We all stood together in the front living room and Bishop Dewi gave his blessing on the house and Trust. All our Trustees, Roger Toms, our builder, and his wife Florinda, as well as Rhiannon, the bishop's wife, together with other old friends and helpers were there.

At the end of the day when goodbyes were being said, Roger shook John's hand: "If you ever want to do another house," he said, "could we build a new one from scratch? It would be cheaper and easier." We laughed; we had no plans to jump through all the necessary hoops again. Two houses was one more than we had ever intended or wanted. We were glad to get back home and relax for a while, and to continue to work to put the Trust on a sound financial base.

CHAPTER 13

Shoulders to the Wheel

'Putting your shoulder to the wheel
when the coach gets in the mud.
That's what I've been doing all my life.'
A Trollope – *The Small House at Allington* (1864)

WHY DID WE embark upon a third project for the Trust? Was it dreamed up one wet Saturday afternoon? Always a vulnerable time for us; we have made some of our more foolish and extravagant decisions/purchases in the doldrums of wet Saturdays. Not for us harmless window shopping, but actual purchase of some furniture, or a new car, or the promise given to do something which in the cold light of workday Monday we wished undone. Was it hubris? Pride in what we had achieved for the Trust leading us to believe we could easily cope with more? Was it the unrelenting rise in the number of families wanting to holiday at Harriet's House and Giltar View that led to John feeling the pressure of being unable to satisfy the need? After a good deal of discussion, the Trustees had decided that each year we would send all the families on our mailing list a provisional booking form asking for their preferred house and choice of dates where possible. In this way we hoped to share the holiday weeks around to give as many families as possible the chance to have a summer school holiday week. Six weeks of school holiday, even doubled, meant that only twelve families could be accommodated. All the forms were prepared, envelopes addressed and posted on the same day. To our dismay, virtually by return of post, the school holiday weeks for the entire year ahead could be allocated. Within a short time both houses were each booked for some thirty weeks of the year. The alternatives were not very satisfactory either. If we allowed families to book for the following year as they left (as happens in most commercial lets), then new families would be at a disadvantage. A waiting list for future years was not satisfactory either, as many of the children involved have life-threatening conditions with uncertain life expectancy.

So, whatever the reason, most probably a mixture of all of these, in early October 1999 John voiced the opinion that we should expand our horizons again. "Let's do what Roger suggested," he said. After completion of the building works at Giltar View, Roger Toms (by now a friend, as well as builder) said that he was tired of pulling old properties apart. If we were to add another property he felt we should tackle a purpose-built new house. In his experience it would be no more expensive and better in the long term.

Realising that we would be unlikely to find a building site within the town, we decided that somewhere between Tenby and Pembroke and no further than five miles from a beach, would suit our needs. John phoned Roger, "If you hear of a building site that would do us – between Tenby and Pembroke, no more than five miles inland, let us know will you?" Roger agreed to keep his eye open and his ear to the ground.

Within 48 hours Roger telephoned us. "You'd better get down here quickly. I've found a good site but it won't be on the market for long." Hastily arranging for a neighbour to look after our cats, we set out the following morning to meet with Roger and view the site. We met him at the Ridgeway, the old road from Tenby to Pembroke. The road up to the Ridgeway is narrow, winding and steep. At the top of the steep hill was the potential building site. It was a fine mild October day. Roger had the details with him:

* Approximately 1¼ acre residential site with detached rundown cottage
* Spectacular views of Tenby town, coastline, Caldey Island and beyond
* Detailed planning consent for the construction of a new dwelling to replace the existing cottage

In the warm autumnal sunshine the site did not give the lie to the estate agent's description. The views across to the sea and coast were indeed spectacular. Caldey Island lay like a jewel in the blue, sparkling water. Looking north, from the top of the paddock next to the cottage site, the Preselli Hills, presumed source of the ancient Blue Stones used by the builders of the Neolithic stone circle at Stonehenge, could be clearly seen. The garden had long since reverted to rough grass and the cottage, which was virtually derelict, stood in the apex of a triangle where the road from Penally came up to join the Ridgeway. A single track road, Strawberry Lane, formed the other side of the triangle. It was almost perfect. Even the presence of a mobile phone mast in the corner of the paddock did not seem much of a problem. That little bubble of excitement began to rise again as we explored the site. There was an old static caravan and a broken-down stone outbuilding in one corner and plenty of junk lying about the garden and along the hedgerow. We went back to Roger's house and talked about the possibilities. We came to the decision to try and secure the site. The asking price was £85,000. The Trust had nothing like enough money to cover the price, but we reasoned that we could remortgage our own house to loan the Trust the purchase price. If we failed to raise sufficient funds within two or three years to complete the project, we knew that we could put the site up for sale again.

In Tenby town the following morning, we put an offer of £78,000 to the agent. He went away and made some phone calls and, much to our surprise, our offer was accepted.

On 19 October we received the notification of sale confirming our purchase of the Wheelabout, subject to contract. The land around the property had formerly been in the copyhold of the Manor of Penally, and the little cottage known as the 'Wheelabout', we understand, was so-called because it stood at the point where the horse-drawn coaches from Pembroke were 'wheeled-about', because the narrow road down to Penally village was too steep for the coach to negotiate safely. The cottage had also perhaps at one time served as an alehouse or pub for the passengers on the coach, although whether or not they then walked down to the village we don't know. So now, the Trust was hoping to acquire a second old pub into its ownership (the first, of course, being Harriet's House on the harbour in Tenby). During the next three months we arranged a mortgage and attended to the various legalities involved until on the 21 January 2000 the purchase was completed with freehold title to the property vested in the Trustees of the charity. Eight years, less one day, after Harriet's death we were all once again setting off on a new adventure.

Whilst waiting for the exchange of contracts on the Wheelabout, we had met with Andrew Muskett, an architectural technologist, with whom Roger had previously worked. He agreed to act as the Trust's architectural technologist and design team leader for the project. That was in early December 1999. Events seemed to be moving very quickly. Andrew began to draw up some preliminary plans based on our schedule of accommodation: in order to maximise the views around the site, we wanted the sitting room upstairs, a platform wheelchair lift to the upper floor, where the special bedroom with tracked ceiling hoist to an en suite bathroom with dished floor would be. There would also be a storage room, dimmer switches in the bedroom and a double bedroom next to it with an en suite shower room for the parents or carers. On the ground floor we asked for a large kitchen/diner, two more bedrooms, and a family bathroom. The house would have to be accessible throughout for a wheelchair. From conversations with families over the years we knew that an accessible heated indoor swimming pool would be an attractive and welcome addition to any 'wish list'. We had already spoken to a supplier who had experience of pools for disabled children. He had told us that the builder could do all the preparatory work. Initial estimates were that the cost of a pool, twenty-four feet by twelve feet with a gentle slope of say two feet eight inches to four feet eight inches deep, including liner and heat exchanger, could be in the region of £15,000. In for a penny in for a pound, we thought. If we are going to do this project, let's make it as good as we can. We asked Andrew if this pool could be in some sort of conservatory-style addition to the main house although we feared that the 'housing element' and necessary extra rooms for a changing facility could prove to be prohibitively expensive.

Andrew set to work and soon produced sketches and plans for the Trustees to see and talk about. He also had preliminary talks with the county planners to ensure that what we wanted would be acceptable. Revised plans, radon gas reports, land survey reports, engineer's inspection of ground conditions: we can follow Andrew's progress through his letters to us. We had no experience or knowledge of any of these matters – but the finalised, approved design gave us everything we had asked for and more.

During that new millennium year we again made an application to the National Lotteries Board in Wales for a grant to cover the cost of building the new house. It seemed to us, a very large amount of money. We felt greatly daring to ask for just shy of a quarter of a million pounds; two hundred and forty-four thousand, seven hundred and fifty-nine pounds. We looked at the amount in both words and figures: £244,759. Would anyone think that our basic simple idea (provision of properly adapted, equipped, accessible holiday accommodation for the disabled) was worthy of backing to such a large amount? Nonetheless, we reasoned that if we wanted the project to succeed we needed substantial backing.

The forms of application were again formidable, but previous experience gave us confidence: costings, business plans, target users, numbers, aims and outcomes, timescale, other sources of funding were all dealt with in order. We find in our records an estimate of costs. It is all there from the estimated fees for the architect, quantity surveyor, land survey, the building construction and drainage to the cost of each piece of special equipment and furniture that would be needed. The pool house, which we had wondered if we could afford, accounted for £37,500. The lift would need just over £11,000. At the bottom of the page is written 'estimated balance to fund £244,759'.

We looked at the types of organizations and projects that had received large grants previously. "I think that our cause and what we want to achieve is as good as anyone's," Kit said (whistling in the dark no doubt). "There's no reason why we shouldn't be given what we ask for."

In the post on 11 August was the longed for letter. Holding our breath, we opened the envelope. Yes and yes again. We were being offered all that we had asked for. The phone was red-hot as John spread the news to all and sundry. We were almost overwhelmed with emotion and excitement. During the late autumn, John and Barrie Jones were invited to visit the Royal Mint at Llantrisant near Cardiff to receive the cheque at a special presentation ceremony – our grant marked the awarding of over £100 million to groups in Wales. John and Barrie were photographed amongst large tubs of coins – a picture which appeared on the front page of the winter edition of the lottery's magazine, together with a description of our project.

The only stipulation of the grant was that the work be put out to at least three tenders and the Trust must accept the lowest of them. Like the Billy Goats Gruff in the nursery rhyme, we expected to skip lightly over that particular bridge. Full planning permission was immediately applied for; we told Roger that he would need to tender for the work and asked Andrew and the quantity surveyor who else might be approached.

Roger was not optimistic about his chances of getting the contract, and thought that a larger firm than his would undercut what his costs would be. We didn't want to contemplate doing the project without him, but, of course, he was proved correct in his assumption.

For the first time the scales tipped slightly from confidence to apprehension, as we accepted the lowest tender from a firm based in Narberth, some ten miles from Tenby. Roger assured us that he would continue to be a friend and supporter but would have to merely watch from the sidelines and not interfere. He and Florinda, his wife, were generous, as always, in offering us friendship and a place to stay on our visits to Tenby. Andrew and the quantity surveyor, Keith Pearce, would be our guides and take responsibility for the proper overseeing of progress. Amongst our Trustees, both Graham Blackburn and Barrie Jones had experience of large industrial project management, so we would be well supported.

And so it started in earnest. The old static caravan on site was to serve as a meeting place. Cramped, dirty and smelly, it was either damply cold or steamily hot with the help of a bottled gas heater. Not ideal, but serviceable. We went to an initial meeting on 2 May 2001. Barrie Jones came from Brecon with us, and Andrew introduced us to Keith Pearce, the quantity surveyor, and a representative from TPT of Narberth, the builders chosen on the basis of their tender being the cheapest, as instructed by the Lotteries Board. The meeting established that, as agreed in the contract, the work would cost £202,524.38. We were becoming used to the sight of the large amounts of money involved. The work was scheduled to begin on 14 May and finish on 4 March 2002. It was agreed that Andrew would monitor and control standards and quality and that all instructions were to be given via him, so that there would be no confusion.

The meeting, having dealt with a variety of other work-related obligations ended with a date fixed for another site meeting on 14 June, in the afternoon. We felt satisfied with how things had gone. The report of the second meeting, which we did not attend, showed that the old building had been demolished, the foundation excavated and ready for the concrete, and that reinforcement was being fixed for the pool. It seemed that a good start had been made.

At the next month's meeting, in the second week of July, we saw that the hole for the pool had been excavated and was ready for the next stage of making the cavity waterproof before a layer of polythene sheeting was put in place prior to the block-work facing. We were interested to see work in progress also on laying the precast concrete beam and block floor. We were assured that the works were on schedule and that there would be no difficulty in completing the work on time. A printout of the programme was promised for our information. As we were leaving the foreman spoke to Kit, saying that on our next visit in a month's time we would be amazed at the amount of progress we would find.

We received the builder's schedule of work four days before a meeting on 21 August. Jo and Graham were with us as we walked around the house-to-be. "Well," said Kit. "I am indeed amazed at the amount of progress they've made, it's virtually undetectable." A month of fine, warm and sunny weather had passed, during which several pillars of a few courses had been erected on the concrete base. The mortar between most of the blocks gleamed wetly showing that they had been laid very recently. It was an inauspicious start to an uncomfortable meeting.

Apologies from the builder for the lack of progress were somehow not entirely convincing. He said that he had had difficulty in getting bricklayers and currently only one team was working on the site. Graham asked if their programme had actually allowed for more than one gang and voiced his concern whether the block-work would be completed during the time allocated on their schedule. Not a problem said the builder. They were only two weeks behind, and had plenty of scope to finish on target. He saw no reason why the building should not be ready for the roof to be put on at the end of September.

"What about putting in the pool and lift?" asked John. "That doesn't appear on your programme. And there's very little time given for landscaping." The builder was conciliatory and agreed to "look into the matter and revise the programme." The meeting ended with a recorded note:

> Client Matters
> 2 Progress:
> Disappointment was expressed at the lack of progress on site. JD/GB stated that this was an important project for the Trust and it must be completed on time. Bookings had been taken from next Easter and there could be no possibility of any overrun whatsoever on the contract period. PT (builder) once again assured the client that every effort would be made during the next month to improve progress, and assured him that the work would be completed on time.

It was a relief when the edgy meeting came to an end. John, with his usual intractable optimism, was busy taking bookings from families and we had to keep pushing the work along. By the end of September, work was still two weeks behind. Graham was not happy and stressed the need for the contractor to make up the lost time.

By the beginning of November work was now about three weeks behind schedule. The autumnal gales of wind and rain had arrived. In such an exposed position, the wind comes in full force from the Irish Sea and the rain is driven almost horizontally so that, at times, it is difficult to remain upright. On one memorable day, Kit had to shelter behind Andrew's comforting bulk and hang on to his coat-tails in order to gain sanctuary in the house. The window frames were late in arriving and, although photographs show that the roof was ready for the slates, the house could not yet be made properly weatherproof.

The field and land around the house and lane were deep in mud and lying pools of rainwater. Despite pleas from Kit not to make a mess of the field, it was covered with heaps of debris, the builders' rejected items and general rubbish. Part of the old hedge-bank had been torn out and a large container had been placed in the field, from where spewed yet more detritus which, on inspection, could not all have come from 'our' house. The light-hearted moments were non-existent and real doubts about the wisdom of the whole undertaking threatened to overwhelm us. Time, perhaps, to leave the worry about what we could not do to those whose job it was to get the work properly completed. We should concentrate on the furniture and fittings and ordering of the remaining special items of equipment. We needed something positive to lift our spirits from the sodden, muddy scene at the Wheelabout.

So what would lift our spirits from the Slough of Despond – otherwise known as the Wheelabout? Morning assembly at Sennybridge Junior School might be just the tonic our jaded spirits needed. Harriet's Trust had been chosen to have the 'collection' money from the children's autumn term harvest festival service. Each year, a different charity was chosen by the children and staff. We had both known the school and village during our working days and had kept in contact with a number of friends and work colleagues there. Off we went in good time to meet the children gathered in the school hall just before 9 a.m.

Kit had been elected to talk to the children and to thank them. Looking at the expectant faces of some 100 five-to-eleven-year-olds as they sat on the floor in front of her, she explained what their £200 would mean to the Trust and tried to get them to imagine what it would be like to be unable to walk, run or talk. Some knew other children with disabilities whilst others wanted to know what we would buy with their money. Kit told them about the swimming pool being built at the Wheelabout. "We'll put your money towards buying a special hoist to help the children get into the water." She described how a sling, from the arm of the hoist supporting a child or adult, could be lowered into the water: "We'll also use a few pounds of your money to buy a rosemary bush for the garden. Rosemary is for remembrance and is a sweet-smelling herb. The children in wheelchairs will be able to smell the rosemary and every time we look at it we shall remember you and your generosity in thinking about those children who are not as lucky as you are."

We were thoroughly enjoying our visit and meeting up again with headmaster, Ashley Richards, and the other teachers. But the morning was far from over, and a bigger surprise was waiting. Ashley told us to have a cup of tea and wait for him while he got the day's learning underway. He soon reappeared. "That pool hoist you want. You haven't bought it yet?" he asked. "We've got one under the stage in the hall. Do you remember when Andrew Lewis had his rugby injury and the village raised the money to buy him a pool hoist so that he could use the swimming pool? When the pool was shut we dismantled the hoist and stored it here. Otherwise the Council would just have thrown it away." Ashley was quite excited. "I'll ask Andrew and the others if you could have it for the Wheelabout pool. If it's any good, it will save you about £2,000."

The sun came out and put his hat on! We felt a lifting of spirits and a feeling of being on home ground. Sennybridge village swimming pool had been built with money raised by the community and was heated with wood fuel from the waste of a local timber yard. The County Council, who had taken over the running of the pool, had decided it was too expensive to maintain and sometime in the early 1990s had closed it down. The dismantled hoist had been under the stage for several years. Barrie Jones and John went to retrieve the pieces and found everything intact. Ashley reported that both Andrew and the villagers were very happy for us to take the hoist, reassemble it and have it properly tested. As so often happens in rural life, there was already a connecting thread between Andrew and Harriet. We had previously met Andrew because Gilly, Harriet's beloved carer, had worked with him after Harriet's death. Indeed somewhere in our memorabilia is a local newspaper cutting about the original Sennybridge village fund-raising for the hoist. There, in the cutting, is a photograph of Gilly and Andrew. The wheel of fate turning a small circle there, we thought. We remembered that Andrew had even been to Harriet's House at Tenby harbour for a holiday.

Christmas came and went – we were now at the beginning of the New Year and bookings for the month of May started to look very close. At the January site meeting, a little progress was reported. The kitchen was ready for the units to be put in, and the lift was to be installed on 28 January – up a small ladder on our mental board game of snakes and ladders. But we went down the next snake lying in wait, because the staircase, front door and large window frames were late in delivery. However, we were moving up the board towards the winning square, and generally the 'contractor was complimented on the standard of workmanship and efforts made to complete the project on programme,' (Graham Blackburn's reservations about the rate of progress notwithstanding).

By February, although bad weather was still hampering outside work, the builder was, as ever, optimistic. We kept pushing hard and no doubt earned ourselves a reputation as the client from hell. On our imaginary board game of snakes and ladders, the ladder of progress leading to 'kitchen units installed' was climbed. John looked at the units and promptly slid down the snake of 'bad workmanship leads to frustration and delay.' The carpenter had clearly not been able to distinguish between white and cream colours, and a number of cupboard panels had been put in back-to-front and the front floor edging strip had been cut into numerous small lengths. John gritted his teeth and arranged for someone he trusted to redo what was necessary, whilst telling the builder that we would deduct the cost from our final payment.

We consoled ourselves back at home with stripping down

and refurbishing table and chairs for a kitchen which, we hoped, would soon be ready. The table had come from Gilly; it had originally been left in a cottage that she had lived in. It was old and large enough for ten people to sit around in comfort, and had been stored in a barn for several years after Gilly had moved to another smaller cottage. "You can have it if you like," she said, "I'd be pleased to think of it being used again. We had some wonderful family meals around it, but I haven't any chairs for you!" The table arrived by horsebox, a favoured rural method of furniture moving. We polished the table's top, which we discovered had been made from old shutters, and then cleaned up the sturdy legs. It looked lovely. We found eight kitchen chairs from the 1960s. These we stripped down and painted to Kit's chosen colour scheme and recovered the old seat pads. After another visit to Cardiff, curtains were chosen and ordered. Harriet's friend, David McFall, was deputed to collect and deliver these to us.

Hand-over day, 4 March, was fast approaching. On arrival at the Wheelabout we could see that it was not going to be 'handed-over' that day, or even that week. The builder said that the still missing glass for the balcony doors would take two or three weeks to arrive. Some tiling and decorating remained unfinished with many other items of work still to be completed, including removing the debris from the field and the provision of topsoil followed by seeding. The builder was adamant that all would be complete within the week.

Hand-over eventually took place on 18 March. We would never have publicly acknowledged that this was, actually, a very good result; privately we knew from tales of horror about many 'new-build' experiences of other people, that our builder had in fact delivered pretty well. A lot of the credit for this we give to Andrew Muskett and his unrelenting attention to the project. Some measure of credit also belongs to Graham and Barrie's persistence at the monthly site meetings. John points out that the less than gentle pressure from Kit, together with an overlay of emotional blackmail inherent in the purpose of the enterprise, must also have played a part. It takes a very stony heart to be able to ignore the needs of disabled children, and we were not afraid to use that card when we thought it necessary. An almost audible sigh of relief came from Narberth as the builder was able to bid farewell to the difficult Davises. Of course, in reality, it was not a final farewell, but our part in the 'build' was over and we were more than content that any remaining matters rested with Andrew and Keith Pearce (the quantity surveyor) to resolve.

We still had plenty to do in the remaining weeks before the first family arrived for a holiday. Garden to be planted, furniture and fittings to be put in place and final cleaning and testing that everything worked properly – we hardly had time to draw breath. As ever, we would need the help of our friends.

Interlude
With a little help from Our Friends

Go out into the highways and hedges
St Luke, 4:23

Angela McFall remembers a day at 'The Wheelabout'

Another escapade in which we ended up to our eyes – or – on our knees.

"Can you help for a day?" asked Mr D. Of course we could! Silly us, we always said anything you want – just shout. As usual, we turned up as requested. As usual, we didn't ask, we just did. As usual, the Davis double act outdid themselves.

"What were the tasks for the day?"

"Would you be kind enough to… move a few tons of topsoil and scrub the tile work all around the swimming pool!

Kindness being our middle name or we're just programmed to obey, we said OK.

Preparation – nil.

Tools – minimal.

Soil task – one wheelbarrow, two spades, one brush.

Swimming pool – (Sgt Major Davis out did herself here) nail brush, rags, washing up bowl, carrier bag stuffed with towels as knee pads.

Top soil – first problem the lads (John & Gethyn) encountered was the fact that this small mountain of top soil had actually been delivered to the lay-by just up from the house – the other side of the lane and wall surrounding the section of the garden requiring said topsoil.

The problem of the wall was thought about first. After searching through various bits and bobs on the building site, a stout enough plank was found to make a ramp for the wheelbarrow.

115

A plan was now forming. Simple. Fill barrow, roll it across lane (easy, it was downhill on this bit of the lane), up the ramp, tip soil into garden. From here the soil could be raked into position.

And so it began. Quite quickly it was evident that this small mountain was bigger than it looked. Four barrow loads didn't even scratch the surface.

Anyway that's what had to be done, so onward. Dig, fill, push, tip. The digging was back breaking. The push up the ramp was hard going – the ramp was steep and bounced under the weight of the barrow. The brush was going to be redundant for hours yet.

Calls for refreshments were frequent, any excuse to rest!

Onward again.

On one downward barrow run to the ramp a local gentleman slowly drove past – he could easily see the daunting task ahead of our two barrow lads. He waved, wished them well – while slowly shaking his head. Whether it was a sign of sympathy or he was convinced they were mad, we'll never know. Anyway off he went on his merry way along the Ridgeway.

Only an hour later he drove back down the road from the Ridgeway. He deliberately slowed down to see how much progress had been made by our intrepid two. What he saw was so shocking that the poor man did a wobble towards the hedge. Thankfully, it was rectified quickly and no damage done. He shook his head, raised his arm and looked suitably impressed. He'd returned just in time to see John and Gethyn brushing up the last little pile of topsoil dust.

Of course, what he didn't know was that our two workers had decided to put brain into gear – brawn was not going to enough. On hearing the sweet sound of a tractor further down the road, they decided to investigate. They found the welcome sight of a JCB with a front bucket. Never let it be said that John does not have the gift of the gab. Some fancy talking, a full explanation of the aims of the charity, and their particular good deed was completed.

Soon the purr of the JCB engine could be heard coming up

Strawberry Lane and that mountain of topsoil was over the wall in a matter of minutes. Well, maybe not minutes, but a heck of a lot quicker than two barrow lads, two spades, one barrow and a brush!

One tractor driver was thanked more than once. He was offered a cup of coffee which was declined as he had to return to his own work task.

John and Gethyn returned to the Wheelabout kitchen looking very pleased with themselves, grinning from ear to ear, and another story to add to the escapades of Harriet's gang. Our commanding officers, Davis and Davis, pleased to knock off another job from the to-do-list.

Meanwhile another David and Goliath task was underway. The swimming pool was complete, beautifully tiled all around. However the grouting was looking dull and not as it should be. It obviously needed a good old-fashioned scrubbing.

While Gethyn and John had been dispatched to the topsoil mountain Angela had been charmed into doing the swimming pool task. Supplies were dutifully found, even the kind thought of, as health and safety for the worker, knee pads (a carrier bag stuffed with old towels).

Creature comforts were improved with the provision of a radio to listen to. So, armed with the washing up bowl, rags and a nail brush, the task started in the far corner.

Does anyone really know how long it takes to scrub around a swimming pool? Does anyone appreciate the wear and tear on a back and a pair of knees? A strategy was set up to do a set number of tiles, change the water in the bowl, stretch all limbs and get rid of the latest crick in the back. I was also able to enjoy the warmth of the sun through those great big windows. I could just spy the top of the topsoil mountain too!

So the time was spent scrub, scrub, stand, change water, scrub, scrub. There were periods of "Is that all I've done?" to "Oh, not so bad, nice patch done!" The knee pad needed shaking on more than one occasion, just to see if there was just one extra inch of soft comfort in there. Fingers needed flexing, there's not a lot to grip on a nail brush. Still the job was getting done. I think everyone thought it best not to disturb the worker, an odd glass of squash came my way and was gratefully drunk.

Landmarks of achievement were met – down one side, along the bottom side, turn the corner and up the other side.

Nearly there… then the door opened – only our dear Kit, showing someone around our wonderful new house! On the threat of one footmark and dire consequences would be handed out, they beat a hasty retreat – after an equally hasty congratulations on a job being well done.

Eventually I made it back to the kitchen HQ to thoroughly enjoy refreshments and a warm glow inside – another task completed.

And the moral of this tale – be very, very careful when you volunteer to our special Davis couple… you never know what it may lead to! We'll never regret our involvement, we've loved every minute. We've made superb friends, had wonderful fun, shared great meals and thought of Harriet every step of the way.

Anne & Mike Chamberlain hedge their bets

As the Trust's third property, The Wheelabout, was nearing completion, it was time for us to make our small contribution. On Saturday, 14 March, 2002 we covered the upholstery in our small motor caravan with bin bags and filled it with plants which Kit had collected for the Wheelabout garden. We also managed to pack in two large metal components for the swimming pool hoist, but couldn't manage the boxes of crockery so they would have to wait for the next trip. The day was bright and we had a very pleasant drive over, spotting two pairs of red kites on the way. We arrived at Penally to find that lots of work was still to be done, and the architect and the builder were in the middle of a deep and, at times, heated discussion. We unloaded the van and crept away!

On the Sunday we were due to collect a large consignment of

heritage hedging plants which a work party from the Pembrokeshire National Park had agreed to plant between the Wheelabout and the road. The hedging was to come from a nursery called Tŷ Rhos Trees, Felindre Farchog, which we knew to be in the lanes near Newport. We thought it would be sensible, this being before the days of helpful things like Google Earth, to locate the right place while we had a bit of time and no deadlines to meet. After a couple of unsuccessful sweeps through the village, we went to the local pub to ask for directions. Once we knew the right small turning to take, we could see that there was a very small sign to Tŷ Rhos Trees in the hedge and we soon found the nursery, a large concern growing a huge variety of native trees and shrubs.

Confident now that we would have no trouble on Sunday morning, we conjectured that we could shorten our return route by following the lanes back south – we had our road map after all, so we should get back to the main road without having to turn around. This turned out to be one of our lesser good decisions! The nursery advertises itself as being 'at the foot of Carn Ingli' and, indeed, as we set off we could see the mountain ahead of us. The lanes we headed down became narrower and more winding and we crossed road junctions with confusing signposts and some with no signposts at all. Through the trees we caught occasional glimpses of Carn Ingli, but it was never where we thought it should be – it was on our right, then our left, then once again ahead! When we passed the same riding stables we had passed just after leaving the nursery, we knew we'd travelled in a complete circle, so admitted defeat.

Sunday was a miserable day, cold and wet. We once more spread the bin bags around in the van, adding a few more for good measure and drove to Tŷ Rhos. The owner was a softly spoken gentleman who gave off a comforting aroma of wood smoke and who wore the most amazing woolly hat, an enormous floppy turban with a rolled edge, knitted in bright red wool. He had the bundles of hedging ready for us, but they were dripping wet and very muddy, so we stacked them in the van with care, trying not to disturb the plastic bags too much. When we thought we had finished, he suddenly produced two large sacks of 'natural fertilizer', otherwise known as manure! We had a very smelly journey back to the Wheelabout and then got a soaking once more as we unloaded the van. The wet weather was, however, just the thing for the new hedge and it has thrived.

CHAPTER 14

On the home straight

'Metaphorically, to be on the home straight
is to be almost home and dry'
Oxford University Press Reference Dictionary

THE WEEKS BETWEEN the hand-over of the finished house
and the arrival of the first family for their holiday sped past
in an absolute blur of activity – friends came and helped with
various tasks and went again. Our goddaughter and mother
came for the day and soon spotted one potential hazard. Sally,
at nine years of age, was lively but petite. "Mummy I'm just
going to the bathroom," she said, "I'll take my mobile with me
in case I can't get the door open, then I can phone you if I
need help." The door closure insisted upon by fire regulations
was so fierce that it was very difficult for anyone, other than a
strong man, to open the door. Kit was relieved to know that she
was not literally losing her grip as she too had found it hard
to open the door. The offending closure had to go. And why
was it, that when the lavatory in the downstairs bathroom was
flushed, sewage floated up via the floor drain, into the wheel-in
shower room on the opposite side of the corridor? The builder
was sent for. We once again held our breath and hoped that
the solution did not include digging up the floors. More sighs
of relief – rubble left in the outside drain was blocking the free
flow of waste. The problem was fairly easy to put right and the
floors remained intact.

Pat Sykes had been appointed to look after the house and families. As with Harriet's House and Giltar View, we had been lucky to find someone with experience of the needs of children and adults with disabilities. Pat seemed to have boundless energy as well as a warm personality. She and Kit received instruction from the 'pool-man' about the mysteries of the pumps, machines, cleaning agents and maintenance needed to keep the pool running at the necessary standard of hygiene. Some long time afterwards, Kit asked Pat a question which had been troubling her. "Did you understand anything we were told that day? He might as well have been speaking in a foreign language for all I could understand. The whole thing frightened the life out of me." Pat admitted that, at the time, she was equally baffled and that at first she would wake in the night worrying about the pool. With numerous phone calls to the 'pool man' for advice and reassurance she gradually became confident. "Well," said Kit, "you certainly hid your feelings very well because I thought you understood it all straight away and it was just me." Kit's inability to understand anything of a technical nature is legendary in our family.

The furniture and curtains arrived and we were given a masterclass in the art of hanging curtains by another friend (who travelled down from Brecon), as he didn't want the windows to be improperly dressed.

At last. At last. Everything was as ready as we could make it. We sat in the kitchen at the family-sized table with the young woman from the National Lottery who had come to have a look at how their grant had been spent. She was very complimentary, but we were slumped in exhaustion. "If we ever, ever, get in touch to say we want a grant to do another house – just shoot me," entreated Kit.

Open day dawned fine and clear. In the early May sunshine, the house and garden, although rawly new, looked welcoming and impressive. More than 60 visitors came to look and comment. The ladies from the Trust's charity shop in Brecon travelled together on a staff outing. Old friends from Llangynidr and Brecon came down and mingled with a number of families who had already holidayed at Harriet's House and Giltar View. They recorded their comments in the Visitors' Book; Jean Dorras was eagerly waiting for 11 May when she and her disabled son Mark would be celebrating their birthdays in our "wonderful, wonderful house". There were a number of wheelchairs testing out the rooms and accessibility during the open day and on the following day, 6 May, the formal, official opening ceremony took place. Harriet's old friend, the Rev. Kelvin Richards, gave a short speech and blessed the house. Dr Sandy Cavenagh spoke to the visitors standing in the garden at the front of the house. Then, once again, the doors were opened to allow everyone in. Harriet's best boys, David and Gethyn McFall were once again in attendance – young adults by now. Whilst the assembled company was enjoying refreshments, John was interviewed by Frank Hennessy on Radio Wales; he had to retreat to a cupboard to do this on the phone because of the noise level in the house.

After the opening, Hazel Cook, Chair of the Pembrokeshire Access Group, wrote to the *Tenby Observer* saying:

> Today in the disabled sector of the community, we set our sights for equality and inclusivity, to put life on an equal par with our able-bodied neighbours.In 'The Wheelabout', both these targets have been met. Here we have yet another jewel in Pembrokeshire's crown, a building to match anything, anywhere.

Ten years after the grief of Harriet's death we were again surrounded and uplifted by friends old and new to help us celebrate her latest achievement.

CHAPTER 15

Down the
Garden Path with Kit

'If you want to be happy for a day get drunk
If you want to be happy for a week get married
If you want to be happy for life become a gardener.'
Chinese Proverb

IN THE HALLWAY of the Wheelabout, just to the right hand side as you come through the front door, hangs a large ornate certificate still in its original frame. Look closely, read the words, and learn that the certificate was presented by the British Order of Ancient Free Gardeners to a Rees Morris of Kilvegy House in February 1917. He was a member of the Begelly Tulip Lodge. From the decorative images on the certificate it is obvious that the Ancient Free Gardeners was a friendly society giving mutual support to its members. John found it in a 'trash or treasure' shop in Tenby and gave it to me because, as he rightly pointed out, not only am I an ancient gardener but I also work for free. When we moved to Pembrokeshire to make it easier to organize the running of the Trust's houses where did we settle? In Begelly, of course.

My father loved to garden and my older sister is an avid gardener, so I suppose it is no surprise that I have spent some of my happiest and most satisfying hours in the past fifty-odd years grubbing about in the soil and plants wherever we have lived. The garden-to-be at the Wheelabout gave me a fresh challenge. An expanse of mud and rubble, leftovers from the building works, to be transformed into a sheltered wheelchair friendly place. It was not going to be particularly easy; exposed to salt winds in the winter gales and rain driven almost horizontally in from the sea, the underlying soil consisting of heavy clay.

Do you, like Harriet, find the whole subject of gardening deeply 'boring'? Are you, like John, wholly ignorant of the matter of plants and soil conditions and fully intend to remain so? If your answer to either of these questions is yes – you may go straight to Chapter 16, if your answer is no – read on!

Andrew, the architect, gave me a scale diagram marked off in squares to help with the design and planting plan. The area in front of the swimming pool sits at the bottom of a gentle rise up to the Ridgeway. Shaped rather like the prow of a ship, it offered the best chance of a sheltered, accessible part of the garden. I asked for a paved area outside the pool house. The upper part of the remaining area was given a retaining wall following the natural slope of the land. A gently sloping ramped walkway could then follow the curve of the wall and around the inner flower bed. When the walls were built, the ship's prow shape was further emphasized.

The first and most important planting would provide a windbreak against the prevailing westerly winter gales. I chose sea-buckthorn and *olearias*, in several different varieties, to form this first defence in the apex of the shape of what I now called the top garden. In early summer the *olearia macrodenta* are full of white flowers. During the winter months orange berries decorate the sea-buckthorn. Hardy fuchsia hedging would continue the screening along the right hand side. Next *phormiums* and *hebes* should be reliably impervious to salt and wind. The remaining space in the top garden would be filled with colourful and fragrant shrubs and aromatic plants. Prostrate rosemary, sage, a rambling rose, campanula, oriental poppies, lambs' ears with their velvety silver grey leaves and lavender-coloured flower spikes – in my imagination I could see and smell it all. The low-walled bed forming the other side of the ramp would have the less hardy plants of ginger lilies or canna lilies, as well as perennial Russian sage which, in summer, is a mass of blue flowers. Sweet peas or other cottage annuals, such as marigolds and love-in-a-mist would fill the gaps. The children could drive their wheelchairs, or be pushed, around the ramp, surrounded by the smell and sight of all the flowers. If I could achieve even a part of my idealised vision, I would be satisfied.

The rubble was cleared, the walls built and several tons of topsoil (pace – John and Gethyn McFall) were applied. Some plants I had grown from cuttings or seed and brought on at home. Others were ordered from nurseries in Cornwall where I had often bought plants for my own garden. My sister brought *pittisporum tenuifolium* seedlings, dug up from her garden in west Cornwall, together with several other offerings. *Pittisporum tenuifolium* is another good wind-resistant plant. It is usually pruned and kept as a shrub, for the black-stemmed young growth and glossy green crinkly leaves are useful in flower arranging. But given time and left unchecked, it will grow into a tree as much as 50 feet tall. It is growing thus at the Wheelabout, mingling with the sea-buckthorns and *olearias*. After nine years it must now measure about fifteen feet in height. I doubt it will ever reach 50 feet, as the wind will prune it and stunt its optimum growth. But in April 2002, working hard and with help from anyone I could persuade to hold a spade or dig a hole, the planting was completed in time for the grand opening. The plants looked small and sparse, and the retaining walls gleamed whitely.

At the back of the house, on the north-facing side, I had chosen a mixture of camellias, varieties of narcissus in abundance, together with *hebes*, *hostas*, *astilbes* and *fatsia japonica*. A clump of golden-oat grass was planted where the slender long stems would be seen from the kitchen window. Next to it a magnolia *stellata*, so that early in the year visitors would see the white star-like flowers that come before the leaves appear.

On the opposite side of the house the garden boundary is marked by a hedge of Pembrokeshire-grown native plants: Hawthorn, Dog-rose, Blackthorn, Field Maple and Guelder rose. (The very plants Mike and Ann went to Tŷ Rhos Tree Nurseries to collect.) Some 90 metres long, the planting area was prepared as part of the community service programme run by the Probation Service. Not only was the ground dug but large stones were removed where necessary. Someone, I forget who, gave us a large sack of mixed daffodil bulbs which one group planted for us along the line of the hedge on the roadside. Stone picking and bulb planting are rather monotonous, back-breaking tasks and may well have encouraged some of the young offenders to reflect upon the wisdom of their past behaviour. The young hedging plants were put in, in pouring rain, by two volunteers from the Pembrokeshire Coast National Park. Facing the big windows of the swimming pool, the hedgerow sits just behind a retaining wall built to accommodate the rise in the land level. Sitting inside, in the steam and warmth of the pool and looking through those big windows, the planting under the hedge on a level with the top of the wall is easily seen. It is also at wheelchair height when going along the path to the top garden. This little narrow planting area is only some 30 feet long, but is one of my favourites. In late winter there are snowdrops underneath the hawthorn and blackthorn. These are gradually increasing in numbers after a hesitant start. The January hedgerows along the Ridgeway have, in places, large shining clusters of snowdrops and perhaps one day the hedgerow that we planted may be similarly adorned. The snowdrops are overlapped and followed by primroses (which I grew from seed) described by the poet John Clare as 'the flowers that truly bring the welcome news of sweet returning spring'. The pale yellow and pink clumps, with their delicate scent always reminds me of an Easter treat which my grandmother sent me for many years. A parcel would arrive from west Cornwall, the contents of which never varied: a packet of Cornish gingerbread biscuits or Fairings, and an old tin with a dented green lid (once used to put school-dinner sandwiches in). Inside, carefully packed in damp moss and tissue, the tin was full of primroses. As the lid opened, the delicate sweet scent of flowers and Cornish air with undertones of moss wafted out. My grandmother had picked these from the fields and hedges on her walk to see friends for afternoon tea; a custom she continued until she was unable to manage the walk – probably in her late eighties. It was an Easter gift that was far better than any chocolate egg.

But back to the Wheelabout garden. Here, under the hawthorn and blackthorn cheerful bright celandines are establishing themselves among small green ivy leaves. Little narcissi and bluebells follow as spring turns to early summer. If you look carefully under the hedgerow, in amongst its newly emerged leaves you can find one of my favourite small, but interesting, late spring plants. The Latin name is worth remembering if you can, because it describes the feature of the plant which makes it memorable: *Arisarium proboscideum*. The Latin word for trunk or elongated nose is proboscis (think of an elephant), so *proboscideum* means having an elongated part. A little spike of tiny flowers is hidden in a hooded, dark brown spathe or bract that is drawn out into a tail of up to six inches long – that's sixteen centimetres to younger readers or visitors to the garden. This little spike of flowers in its brown hiding place emerging amongst the green leaves, looks just like the tail of a mouse and so its common name is, naturally, the mouse plant. It is a little curiosity which never fails to amuse and delight.

The part of the garden in front of the house and overlooked from the dining room and upstairs sitting room windows is the most exposed and open area. The driveway is bordered on one side with grass, where ball games can be played in safety. On the far side the prevailing westerly winds shred the edges of the *phormium* leaves and a *cordyline* already leans drunkenly towards the boundary fence. On windy days clothes, hung out to dry, tug and billow on the washing line as if about to take flight over the trees and down the hill to Penally village. In early summer, the grass is starred with white daisies and yellow dandelions. Fancifully, I think of this as our modern version of a fifteenth-century jewel garden, where brightly coloured flowers were planted in the formal grassed areas. I remember seeing a re-creation of this sort in the cloister garden at Aberglasney, near Carmarthen. Our dandelions and daisies are multiple in number and haphazard in design. Nothing formal about this, but I am always sad when the mower dispatches them in order to keep the grass useable for playing on.

Later in the creating of the garden and, once again, with the help of the Probation Service, two more beds were dug out to finish my scheme. The young men worked hard and did a good job in preparing the soil. Another hardy fuchsia hedge was to give some shelter to a 'hot' bed of *montbretias* and grasses. The *montbretia*, in a range of orange, yellow and red shades, mingling with red-hot pokers, day lilies and ornamental grasses, give late summer colour and movement. This bed was not fully finished until well after the opening of the house by which time I had the benefit of cheerful, energetic and knowledgeable help from Jenny Axon.

I have discovered that when ladies who garden (as opposed to ladies who lunch) reach a certain maturity, well-meaning friends advise engaging a retired man or pensioner to help with the heavier work. Rubbish, I say! What is needed is someone young and energetic, with strong knees and wrists. What I don't want is some old boy who thinks gardening is all about straight lines, bedding plants and growing vegetables in rows. Compatibility of garden philosophy is nearly as important as strong wrists and knees. I'm with the seventeenth-century poet, Robert Herrick, who wrote that:

A sweet disorder in the dress
Kindles in clothes a wantonness.

In the garden also a little 'sweet disorder', some natural mix of self-seeding, planting that is not too ordered and constrained do, as Herrick said, 'more bewitch me, than when art / Is too precise in every part'. Jenny and I share a very similar philosophy – essential in a gardening buddy. Not too much regimentation, a wait and see approach with a liking for the occasional adventure in gardening by growing something new from seed, just to see what happens.

Just before the opening of the Wheelabout, even a cursory look at the guest list showed that space for car parking would be a problem. No public transport runs along the Ridgeway, and the lanes leading up from the village are steep and narrow with nowhere suitable to leave a number of cars. Jenny had a plant nursery just two fields away and agreed to play car hostess to visitors on the day. Parking along the top of her drive – in the nursery enclosure together with the top of our field and the lay-by (where the never-to-be-forgotten top-soil mountain had been dumped) we were satisfied we could cope. In no time at all Jenny was enlisted into Harriet's troop. She agreed to help with the garden and over the next six or seven years bore the brunt of the hard work, often bringing with her a young lad, David, as her assistant. So now we had a little team working away to nurture and maintain the garden.

During the first years in the life of the garden the planting flourished. Mild winters allowed us to grow a number of more tender plants. Dark leaved canna lilies with orange flowers grew five or six feet tall giving dramatic emphasis to the bed beside the front patio. My favourite though was the *echium pininana*. I had seen this growing in west Cornwall and was determined to try raising some from seed. Two packets of seeds arrived via the Chiltern Seed catalogue (obligatory bedtime reading for the unreconstructed seedaholic) and proved surprisingly easy to germinate and bring into growth. When they were large enough we planted them in the ramped garden and when fully grown the flower spikes, rising to a majestic twelve or fifteen feet above the large rough leaves, made everyone walking past stop to look and wonder. Small blue flowers, about the size and colour of forget-me-nots, covered every inch of each tall spire; all summer long they sang as numerous visiting bees hummed and searched for nectar. Butterflies too were attracted to the show-stopping group. When the flowers faded and the plants died back, we collected the small hard seeds and the life cycle started again,

For a number of years the *echiums* flourished and gave a subtropical air to the ramped garden. In their native Canary Islands *echiums* are true biennials – growing from seed in their first year and flowering in the second year before dying. They are frost hardy to about minus five degrees centigrade, if growing in a fairly sheltered spot. The seed we gathered in the late summer was sown immediately and germinated quickly. The young plants nurtured in a warm greenhouse during their first winter and then were planted out the following summer before they grew too big to transplant. Then, alas, for three years running winter temperatures in south Pembrokeshire fell to lows inhospitable to *echiums*. In 2010, in a more prolonged cold period, the road up to the Wheelabout was impassable with snow and ice. In the bitter cold the *echiums*, together with a number of other tender plants were killed off, leaving bare places in the garden. I think all gardeners regret the loss of favourite plants but, nevertheless, I equally always enjoy choosing something new. With luck we may be able to grow *echiums* again if the cold winter cycle does not go on for too long.

A garden is never static and each year yields its mixture of satisfaction and frustration; each year I vow will be my last to buy seed or spend hours pruning, digging, mulching and weeding. But, of course, it is that very changeability that keeps us in thrall and, when springtime arrives, the siren call of the garden is too strong to resist and off I go again. I am lured on by the hope that in May the oriental poppies will bloom brightly, that their silky delicate petals will not rot in the bud or the flowers be spoiled by rain too soon after opening; perhaps this year the albertine rose will not be smothered in greenfly or blackspot, will the hostas withstand the monster slug attack...? The garden path winds on and I carry on along it unable to resist the tantalising prospect of garden dreams fulfilled. What did Alexander Pope write?

> Hope springs eternal in the human breast
> Man never is, but always to be blest

I wonder if he was a gardener as well as a poet?

An Interlude with Herbie

Herbie was born in a large block of Forest of Dean stone. Under the skilled hands of Catriona Cartwright – a young woman working with stone in her studio near Hay-on-Wye – Herbie took shape. A dragon recumbent, sleepily lying along the front wall of the ramped garden, guarding the children against harm. "I couldn't stop him from smiling," explained Catriona, when she and her husband brought Herbie to the garden. "The children called him Herbie, because he only eats plants." So Herbie he remained.

His grey coloured head with its hooded eyes and smiley mouth lies along one end of the curved wall, close and low enough to be touched by children starting up the ramp. A steel spike driven into the wall ensures that he cannot topple over or take off in flight. Along the curve of the wall his spines lead round to his tail, curled at rest. A mixture of ivy plants give Herbie his coat of green scales. He is ageing gracefully; lichen is beginning to establish on his head and tail – and the ivy has almost covered his back.

Set in the pavers between Herbie and the outside door of the swimming pool is a carving of a Celtic knot, the eternal circle of friendship and love. On the wall nearby, carved on slate in fine cursive script by Catriona, are Harriet's words: "Time can come like a wind."

CHAPTER 16

Tales from the Cellar

'I came upstairs into the world;
For I was born in a cellar.'
William Congreve – *Love for Love* (1695)

WE CUT OUR fund-raising teeth with the Research Trust for Metabolic Diseases in Children (now metamorphosed into CLIMB or Children Living with Inherited Metabolic Diseases). This charity, established in 1982 by Peter and Leslie Greene, has grown into an umbrella support and fund-raising charity for families with children affected by any one of some 2,000 inborn errors of metabolism such as Leigh's disease which Harriet had. The charity also supports and encourages research into the causes and possible treatments of metabolic disease.

In 1983 we formed the south Wales branch for this Trust and started out on the fund-raising path. Looking back from a distance of some 28 years, we marvel at our energy and determination to combine looking after Harriet and fund-raising. A balloon race, choir concerts, arranging for runners to take part in the London and Cardiff marathons, visiting schools to receive donations raised from children, were but a few of the activities. We were continually amazed and encouraged by the support of friends and strangers. We look back at our collection of newspaper cuttings and photographs and exclaim at how young we all looked and at the number and variety of events that we either arranged or benefited from. Some of the faces in the photographs are now just that – names now sadly forgotten. Others we have lost touch with but remember with affection – and others have become and remain close friends.

During the early 1980s charity shops were in no way as prolific or such big business as they are now. We progressed from the usual nightmare, otherwise known as jumble sales, to pop-up shops. With relief we no longer had to face the line of avid bargain hunters waiting outside the village or community hall when they rushed through the doors, advancing like locusts towards the tables piled high with jumble (scenes repeated nowadays at January sales time). Instead we beguiled the owners of empty shop premises in Brecon to allow us to use them for perhaps a week at one time. Then, in 1987, a very small shop, tucked away in a narrow side street of Brecon town, became vacant.

After some discussion, we decided that we would take on the lease in John's name coupled with his friend and fellow Lion, Barrie Jones. The plan was to continue to fund-raise for RTMDC and a shop would be less work than continually trying to organize pop-up shops. Certainly this was a fine example of fools rushing in, the bliss of ignorance or any number of similar adages that come only too readily to mind. Add to this dire prophecies of various doomsayers: "A charity shop? In Brecon? That's not going to work! Nobody will support a permanent charity shop. Who's going to staff it?" and so on. We needed to keep our resolve and belief that we were doing the right thing.

We went to view the shop. The large front window was running with condensation. Once inside the smell of damp was strong. It was an inauspicious start. A narrow low-ceilinged staircase led down to the cellar. It was ill lit, with plaster on the walls in one corner looking soft and discoloured with rising damp. There was a partial wall across the room with an old sink positioned against it on the further side. Facing the sink behind an ill-fitting door was a lavatory – obviously leaking onto the beaten earth floor. No heating. There was also some old carpeting, folded over and harbouring who knew what lethal germs within its damp heap. John McFall and Barrie put down a damp-proof membrane and a concrete floor, which we painted with grey floor paint. Barrie recalls that his most abiding memory of this was the large number of journeys he made up and down the awkward staircase. The lavatory was fixed, and cleaned thoroughly – as was the sink. John and Barrie fixed up some racks and we were given a number of metal baskets meant for displaying rolls of wallpaper. These fitted onto the racks so that we had somewhere to store clothes and other items as we sorted them out. Angela McFall presented us with a large dehumidifier and we brought an oil-filled electric radiator from home. Once the shop upstairs had been cleaned and decorated, we were almost ready for business. We had the name of the charity put across the window – now we had achieved a double distinction – the first (and at that time the only) charity shop to open in Brecon, and the first and only shop for RTMDC.

Welsh rugby star Cliff Morgan came and declared the shop officially open. He was not the only illustrious visitor to the shop. In 1989, the Duchess of Westminster, as patron of the Research Trust for Metabolic Diseases in Children came to see what we were achieving. It was an occasion both formal and informal. Easy to chat to, she met our volunteers as well as the mayor of Brecon, Geoff Harding, who was also a member of the same Lions Club as John and Barrie. After lunch at the nearby Castle of Brecon hotel, Barrie presented the Duchess with a cheque for £10,000 for RTMDC. Harriet came with Gilly Lawrie so that they could be part of the celebration and another young boy, Tony Gibbs, who also had a rare and awful metabolic condition, came with his mother from Caersws in north Powys. Leslie Greene, as founder of the research trust came from Nantwich to complete the party. John, of course, was quite at ease arranging such an occasion as he had, in the past, been involved with arrangements for royal visits in connection with his work with the Duke of Edinburgh's award scheme. We continued to give money raised from the shop for just over five years, giving in total in excess of £26,000. Following Harriet's death in 1992 and the founding of the Holiday Trust in her name, we decided that we couldn't fundraise for both. As the shop was leased to John and Barrie, it was an easy matter to change the name on the shop front, though it was with reluctance that we had to stop our efforts for RTMDC. Altogether, between 1983 and 1992, we had raised approaching £70,000 for the research trust. But back to the start of our shop-keeping careers.

Word about the shop spread through the town and nearby villages. Volunteers, mostly Brecon ladies of a certain age, offered their services and the stock rolled in. The cellar loomed large in our lives as the endless stream of black sacks arrived to be sorted. Kit became expert at rag-picking, quickly deciding whether or not something was fit for resale. At home, after Harriet was asleep and the night nurse had arrived, the living room floor would be covered with sacks and piles of clothes as Kit sorted quickly through some of the offerings. The metal baskets were then filled and taken back to the shop with their load of clothing that had passed the nose and eye tests and had been priced for sale.

Two of our early customers were Sylvia and big Helen (to distinguish her from little Helen). They told us that they would spot our car going past their houses en route to the shop and would hurry after in order to check on possible bargains. Later, they both became volunteers and joined the sack-sorting team. The cellar would echo with cries and comments as particularly good or ghastly donations were discovered. "Fancy giving that away, it's hardly been worn" or "look at this, the shop price is still on it!" Always tip the contents out onto the table first – never put your hand into the sack was the rule of the day. Sometimes a sack would be opened and quickly tied up again as a malodorous gust of mothballs (or worse) hit the air. On one, never to be forgotten occasion Sylvia, in a moment's abstraction, put her hand into a freshly opened sack. With a loud shriek of horror she cried, "It's a dead cat or something."

But of course it wasn't. Just an old 'dead' fur coat. We sold many fur coats, both real and fake.

The dehumidifier and oil radiator worked well in tandem. Neither was ever switched off during the sixteen years that we had the shop. The cellar became warm and dry and it was surprising how many 'visitors' found their way down the awkward staircase to perch, either on the bottom step or on a heap of sacks to chat, gossip, or unburden their worries and woes. With the low ceiling and warmth, it had something of the air of a confessional that seemed to encourage the urge to talk. One such visitor was Gareth-of-India; he was known to everyone by this soubriquet because he spent as much of his time as he could living amongst the Tibetan people in northern India. He was an excellent photographer and had a fine photographic record of his life there. He would bring some of these down to the cellar and sit and relate his difficulties in getting visas, or travel arrangements. An independent character, his life seemed to be full of incident, adventure and misadventure. He was always on the lookout for unwanted typewriters to carry back to his Tibetan friends.

The road outside the shop was narrow; no room for one car to overtake another, so most of our stock was delivered hurriedly. John appeared at the top of the stairs with two full bin bags – "A very smartly dressed lady had just left these, so it should be good," he called down to the sorters of the day. Alas, no. One man's treasure is another man's trash. Unwashed underwear, stained and torn outerwear, and worn out shoes definitely come into the trash category. On another occasion a young woman threw a large quantity of men's good clothing in through the door, whilst saying: "He's left me, so you can have his stuff!"

Up the stairs, into the world and the shop, the ladies were in control. They were nearly all born and bred locally and, between them, must have known almost every inhabitant of the town and some of the nearby villages – an endless source of local knowledge and gossip. A spare stool beside the counter was usually occupied by a succession of friends and acquaintances and the chat flowed freely between them and customers. We often said that if the shop had been big enough to have a table and chairs for coffee, some would have stayed all day. Each volunteer had her own circle of customers and enjoyed different aspects of her time in charge. Brenda-the-Window is still remembered for her pleasure in arranging goods for sale as she had an unexpected talent for window-dressing. Problems arose when somebody wanted to buy an article displayed, because then it would spoil her arrangement. Each year for the Brecon Jazz Festival a window-dressing competition was held when all the local shopkeepers would vie for the best jazz-themed display. We occasionally tried our hand at this and once even managed to win the first prize. This was due to the artistic creativity of Barrie's two daughters who were delighted to have the chance to indulge their talents. Most of us, however, were content if the window display was constantly changing, because it meant that the sale of goods was brisk.

And so the years rolled on. Our customer base was a mixture of the older generation, whose days were sometimes long and who enjoyed the chat; the unemployed and economically frugal, who did not have much money to spare; the mentally fragile who liked to share their worries and, of course, farmers' wives on market day, looking for serviceable work clothes. There was the man who was going to a wedding and asked the ladies for a complete outfit of suit, shirt, tie and shoes. Amid much hilarity he was kitted out, having made a good contribution to the morning's take. Once Kit was in the cellar sorting sacks when one of the ladies came down to consult. "There's a chap upstairs who wants us to give him a pair of trousers, jacket and shirt. He says he's unemployed, got a job interview in Hereford. He can't afford some decent clothes and the fare to Hereford." Kit went up to have a word. She agreed to give the outfit. The lady in charge that day wasn't too sure. "What if he's telling lies?" she asked. "Well," reasoned Kit, "if he's on the level, then we probably will have helped him a lot. If he's lying we won't have lost much money (about £15). If that's the most I am ever cheated of, then I shall count myself fortunate." We were not however without those who would shoplift, if given half a chance.

We believe that we cornered the market for Mills and Boon paperback books. Kit once counted 300 titles in stock. We were almost embarrassed to charge for them as some ladies returned them, when once read, and then bought some more. It was almost a lending library. Jams, pickles, dried flowers, fresh plants and seedlings were supplied in season by June Lawson and Kit. As one satisfied customer said, "not only can you buy the plant – you get a gardening lesson about it at the same time!"

In time other charities began to open shops in the town, but they made little impact upon us. Our place in the affections of local people was secure. We alone had a rail of children's clothes and, although we gained little profit from their sale, we felt it was important to support young families if we could. One young woman, Mrs Woodhead, was a regular customer for her three children and she and her husband later moved with their family to France to live. Every New Year she still sends a very generous donation to the Trust; the 'collection' money from a carol service held for ex-pats in the French town where she lives. "I was able to clothe my children from your shop. When they were little we had very little money and I was very grateful for your shop, now I want to give something back," she wrote in explanation.

By 2005 a combination of several factors led us to shut up shop: our team of ladies was getting older; the stock market had been moved to an out-of-town site and a supermarket built on the original site. The effect on the end of town where our shop was located was almost dramatic. The farmers' wives no longer came into town and the Friday market in the covered market hall, which backed onto the street where we were, became very run down. Our shop income decreased as our end of the town became more isolated. Plans to shut off the end of the street where a new town by-pass road was to be built, settled the matter. We had decided that the time had come for us to move to Tenby to continue looking after the properties (now three in number and a fourth planned). Like our team of shop ladies, we were getting older and finding it difficult to juggle so many different activities in two places some 80 miles apart.

We were all sad to clear everything away and shut the door of the shop for the last time, but we all had 16 years of memories to look back on. "Where did you buy that?" The question still floats in the ether, "Oh, you know. From that little boutique in Castle Street." "Where?" "Harriet's shop of course!"

CHAPTER 17

Into the Lions' Den

'But it is pretty to see what money will do.'
Samuel Pepys' Diary (21 March 1667)

HAVING AGREED TO purchase Upper Albion from David Manby and set in motion the establishment of a charitable trust, we needed to raise a large amount of money rather quickly. The charity shop was providing the seedcorn but would never attain the sum needed for the purchase, adaption and furnishings required. Then of course, as families learnt about the Trust and what it was providing, more funding was needed when we decided to provide a second house, Giltar View, then a third, The Wheelabout, to meet the demand. In the beginning a major source of income was provided by the Lions Clubs International Foundation. This was achieved through the good offices of Bill Jones who was a member with John of the Brecon Lions Club. Bill was a long-serving and well-respected member of the Lions and this was reflected in the fact that he had been elected to be the chairman of the council of governors of the Lions Clubs of the United Kingdom and Ireland. He was a former bank manager and nicknamed by some of the club members 'Captain Mainwaring' who he resembled in stature, although not in manner. Bill suggested to John that if the Brecon club supported the appeal and this was backed by other clubs in the district, then an application for funding could be made to the International Foundation. The members of the club knew all about Harriet and readily agreed to give their support and made a very generous donation to the fund. Having got the support of his fellow Lions in Brecon, John began a speaking tour of the clubs in the Lions district 105W, covering south Wales and part of south-west England, using Harriet's story and the need for the special holiday accommodation as the basis of his talk. Throughout the tour he was supported by Barrie Jones, also a member of the Brecon club, who had agreed to become the chairman of the Trust.

Lions clubs vary in size of membership which is drawn from all sections of the community. They all share the same objective which is to help those less fortunate than themselves. John and Barrie were greeted and very warmly received as fellow Lions at each club meeting, which was usually preceded by a dinner, pleasing Barrie as he always had, and still has, a good appetite. All the clubs visited were very receptive to the idea of specialist holiday houses for families with disabled children and all were generous in giving financial support. The application then had to go for approval by the Lions district cabinet, where it received unanimous backing. The members of the cabinet were especially pleased to give their support, not only because they saw the application's merit, but because few ideas for funding from the International Foundation had emanated from the district in recent years. Bill Jones saw the application through the council of governors with a recommendation for approval to LCIF at the Lions' headquarters in America. This resulted in a grant of £16,300 being approved. This gave a very welcome boost to our fund-raising and the support of so many clubs lifted our spirits.

After Harriet's House was opened we had a visit from the foundation's international president, Lion James T Coffey, who hailed from Ohio and was making a visit to the UK.

When it came to financing Giltar View, Bill Jones suggested that a second application should be made to LCIF. By now the Trust was well known throughout the Lions district 105W and John wrote to them all. This resulted in more speaking engagements and more dinners. The success of the first house had proved the need, and the Lions were pleased to back a winner. Twenty-one clubs gave wholehearted support, and a second grant of £21,000 was made by LCIF. The Lions Clubs International Foundation development director, on a visit from America, came to Giltar View with representatives of the district and clubs to present the cheque. He said: "This is a project that Lions all over the world can rightly be proud of and a concept which would be marvellous to see in many other places."

The work of the Trust was one of only three charities highlighted in a Lions video showing the type of project supported the organization and, in 1997, earned first prize in the Lions World Bank of Ideas awards. The plaque awarded to the Trust is proudly displayed in Giltar View.

In total the Lions organization has supported the Trust with in excess of £70,000, living up to its motto 'We Serve'.

We made many good friends among the clubs that supported us and were pleased to show them over the houses on their visits to Tenby. Bill Jones is sadly no longer with us, but Sandy Cavenagh and Barrie Jones still serve the Trust as president and chairman respectively. Colin Duncan, another Brecon Lion, together with other members of the club was always ready to assist with the many fund-raising events that we held.

CHAPTER 18

A Dramatic Interval

'All the world's a stage'
William Shakespeare (1564–1616) – *As you like it* (1623)

IT WAS THE autumn of 1992 and we were in Penzance, west Cornwall, staying with Kit's sister Joan. We had not been able to travel so far for some years, and Joan and her husband had not long moved down to Cornwall. Harriet's Trust was officially established and we were enjoying a short break from fund-raising to buy the property on the harbour in Tenby.

Joan told us that she had promised that one evening we all go to see a musical drama about the lives of Ira Sankey and Dwight Moody. The play was to take place in a big Methodist chapel at Stithians, some twenty miles from Penzance. The large chapel building seemed out of proportion to the size of the village, and we wondered where an audience would come from. Our cousin, Tony Jasper, was touring the country with his small company of actors performing the drama, *Feel the Spirit*, which he had written. An only child, he had grown up living opposite Kit's maternal grandmother in Penzance at the very tip of south-west Cornwall. His mother was related to Kit's father and he spent many hours in Granny Francis's, where Kit stayed during every school holiday after her family moved back to Kent at the end of World War II. John still remembers that, barely a month after our wedding, he was left to fend for himself for two weeks in the school summer holidays as Kit hurried down to Penzance 'to make sure that granny is alright.' Even as a very old lady. Granny was mentally alert and interested in modern life and young people. Anthony still talks about her with great affection, and says that on Sunday evenings they would listen together to the programme of hymn singing on the wireless which she loved to sing along with. Radio Luxembourg was another favourite. It must have been then that his love of singing, and hymns in particular, was born. This developed into a committed Christian faith and an impressive knowledge of religious history. In his book, *Moody and Sankey – feel the spirit*, Tony refers to this time spent with Granny Francis, and how the songs that he sang with her was one of the ways he first came to know the work of Sankey and Moody. Although during Harriet's lifetime we had somewhat lost touch, we knew, via the family grapevine, that he was successfully writing and publishing work of a religious nature.

We went off to Stithians, not really knowing what to expect. We knew that Dwight Moody was a nineteenth-century American evangelist and Ira Sankey was his musical partner. From our childhood we remembered singing many hymns from their book, *Sacred Songs and Solos*, but knew nothing about their lives. Joan said that the singers and actors in Tony's small company, the Jasperian Theatre, were all professionals; but it is sometimes difficult to believe that someone you have known since childhood, growing up, felt affection for or been irritated by, been both kind and unkind to, could develop a recognised talent for writing about and promoting the gospel.

At the chapel we sat upstairs in the front row of the gallery looking down on the simple stage setting – just a table and some chairs placed before the imposing pulpit. The chapel was almost full – where had everyone come from? But when the music started we stopped wondering as we were swept along in delighted surprise. The singing and music was wonderful, the acting excellent and the story of Sankey and Moody's life as it was played out before us was, at times, lively and funny and at others, deeply moving. The words and tunes of the hymns were all familiar: 'Blessed Assurance', 'When Peace like a River', 'Ho my Comrades' and 'Shall we gather at the river?' The audience was invited to join in the refrain of some of the songs – which we all did lustily. During the interval Kit remarked on how almost shocked she had been at her first sight of Tony, looking so much like her father in stature, further emphasised by Tony's costume for the part of Moody – a plain black jacket and trousers with a white shirt, just as father had always worn. At the end of the performance everyone applauded heartily; looking up at the gallery Tony had an almost equal shock to see us all looking back down, as Joan had not told him that we were coming.

A little while later Tony told us that he wanted to do something towards our fund-raising and suggested that he would give a benefit performance for the Trust and also invite donations from audiences at other venues on his next tour planned for 1993. And so it was that in November 1993 we found ourselves taking part in a theatrical experience as hosts to the Jasperian Theatre Company. There were six actors, the musical director and accompanist and a stage manager. They arrived in an assortment of vehicles and for a week we were carried along on a tide of enthusiasm, laughter and drama, both on and off the stage. We remember their names and personalities with great affection: Peter Bye, a skilled and experienced musician; Jade Louise Johnston, Fiona Timothy, Ian Farthing, Catherine Fish, Fiona Dunn, Sara Orrell and, of course, cousin Tony. We had persuaded several friends in the village to offer sleeping accommodation to some of the cast and we were to provide breakfast and other meals for each day in which they were with us.

Llangynidr village hall was full to capacity for the special benefit performance for Harriet's Trust. After it was over and the enthusiastic applause had died down, we had the chance to introduce all the players to some of our friends and supporters. June Lawson and Adele Jones from the 'top village' helped us greatly, supplying food, transport and good company during the week-long tour. On the last evening, June gave one of her legendary suppers. Everyone sat basking in the warmth before a fine wood fire in the large fireplace of the old cottage's sitting room. Originally part of the cottage had housed the village blacksmith's forge, and the heat of those forge fires had obviously been absorbed into the spirit of the cottage.

November is not the kindest or warmest month in which to drive about the byways of Powys in the dark evenings. Scattered widely over the county, the venues we had arranged were all in old chapels or churches, not the cosiest of places on winter evenings. But the young actors were very hardy and coped well when the heating was somewhat inadequate or the makeshift dressing rooms chilly and without any creature comforts. At one venue Kit wondered why the audience chose to sit well back from the pews nearest the pulpit and stage set. She remembers deliberately sitting forward to be cheerleader and encourage others to follow. After sitting in splendid isolation until the interval in the drama, she says she had to admit defeat and retreat to a back pew. What the regulars knew about, and we didn't, was the icy blast of a draught that blew at neck level in that part of the building. But whatever the chill of the buildings, nothing could detract from the warmth of welcome we were given at each place and the generosity shown in the provision of refreshments and the giving of donations to the Trust from the audiences.

We got to know our guests and experience at first hand both the angst and fun of being a small temporary part of a touring theatre company. Early in the week Catherine Fish provided an off-stage dramatic crisis when she had to be hastily taken to the eye hospital at Hereford, some 40 miles away. There she was treated for iritis, a painful and potentially serious eye condition. Well-dosed with painkillers, she was the embodiment of 'the show must go on', performing as Mrs Moody (junior) while sporting a jaunty black eye patch, which gave her a faintly piratical appearance. At the end of each evening, winding down over a communal meal at home, we got to know our guests better. Jade, whose singing of 'Blessed Assurance' was a show-stopper, was to be married to a Baptist minister with whom she sometimes arranged to be met when there was a break in the tour. She painted a picture of an attractive, dark haired, young woman, waiting in a convenient lay-by to be picked up by a man (of the cloth). Catherine Fish, who we had often heard singing on the Daily Service on Radio Four, was also an experienced stage performer. We learnt that Peter Bye, the musical director and accompanist, had worked with many famous singers, including Cliff Richard. His arrangements and accompanying of the songs in 'Feel the Spirit' showed just how talented he was. All the young people were fully committed to their task and we thoroughly enjoyed their conversation and laughter and we were sorry when it was time to say goodbye. They signed a programme for us: "Oodles of love" (Ian Farthing); "Lots of love and thanks" (Fiona T); "Thanks for a lovely week" (Sara Orrell); "Great place for a holiday" (Kate Fish). Jade wrote that it was "a good place for a honeymoon." "With great ~~affliction~~ affection," recorded Peter Bye! While Fiona Dunn's message was "and now to lose the weight."

In November the following year, the old wooden village hall in Llangynidr was again filled with the joyous sounds and drama produced by the Jasperian Theatre Company. The story being told was that of William and Catherine Booth, founders of the Salvation Army. Once again we found ourselves hosting the cast. The actors were different but Peter Bye was the musical director and accompanist again. This time, after performing in Llangynidr and Abergavenny, we all trooped down to Tenby. Friends there were generous in providing beds to sleep in and Harriet's House on the harbour was the headquarters. The congregation of St John's Church in the town supported the performance in the church. With another successful occasion under our fund-raising belts, we waved goodbye as the actors drove off to their next venue in Swansea.

By 1995 cousin Tony had added another drama to his

repertoire. Where he got his energies from was a source of wonder. Not content with arranging tours, acting, finding a new casts for each tour, he was also finding time to write. *Glory! Glory! Diolch Iddo!* [Thanks be to Him] was the title of the next drama which he brought to Llangynidr. In the programme for this production Tony wrote:

> This is the third production from the Jasperian Theatre. *Glory! Glory! Diolch Iddo!* continues my aim to explore the world of major Christian figures in drama and music. Our first production was *Feel the Spirit* – it focused on the world of D L Moody, preacher and evangelist and his accompanying singer, Ira D Sankey. Then came William and Catherine, the Booths. This centred on the Booth's setting up a new form of Christian witness in London's East End and from which came the Salvation Army. Billy Bray, the glad man, often called the madman by his detractors, and Evan Roberts at the centre of the young people who led the Welsh revival of 1904–5 bring another powerful story and like the other two, it is well felt and expressed in the music of the heavens.

The old village hall in Llangynidr had been replaced with a splendid large new building. Although bigger and, we felt, somewhat lacking in the intimate atmosphere of the wooden hall, we had assembled a good audience. We were invited to sing the songs either in Cornish (for Billy Bray), Welsh (for Evan Roberts) or English (which most of us monoglots had to do). Probably more Welsh was heard as the company toured the Welsh countryside. Tony obviously enjoyed the part of his fellow Cornishman, Billy Bray. Jeremy Lloyd-Thomas, with impeccable Welsh origins, gave a much acclaimed performance as Evan Roberts.

As with all his productions Tony gave programme space to information about Harriet and the Trust. Money still came to us from his tours, although this was the last performance that we were involved in in Llangynidr. Between the years 1993 and 1998 Tony raised some £12,000 for the Trust, at a time when we were really just at the beginning of its work, and we will always be grateful to him and everyone who 'put money in the plate' for us. We sometimes went and spoke to audiences during the interval time and thus spread the information about the Trust to more and more people.

But most of all our time with the Jasperian Theatre Company experience has given us a store of vivid memories, which are often recollected when we talk about our 'life after Harriet' and how she has changed our lives forever. "Do you remember when…?" we ask when meeting up with old friends as we reminisce about the past. Perhaps Tony will one day write about his experiences of touring with a small company of actors with all the attendant anxiety, fun and adventure that we were able to have a small share in for those few years.

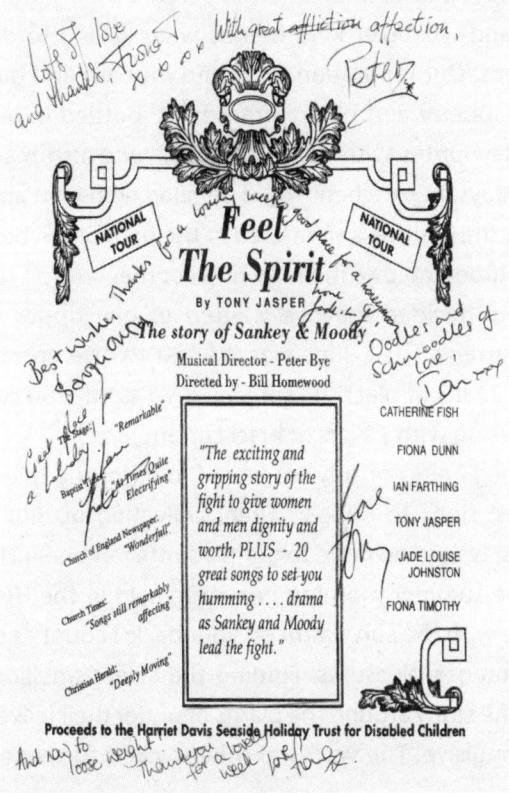

Feel The Spirit

BY TONY JASPER

The story of Sankey & Moody

Musical Director - Peter Bye
Directed by - Bill Homewood

"The exciting and gripping story of the fight to give women and men dignity and worth, PLUS - 20 great songs to set you humming . . . . drama as Sankey and Moody lead the fight."

CATHERINE FISH

FIONA DUNN

IAN FARTHING

TONY JASPER

JADE LOUISE JOHNSTON

FIONA TIMOTHY

Proceeds to the Harriet Davis Seaside Holiday Trust for Disabled Children

Interlude
Kit and June in a Jam

'Jam tomorrow and jam yesterday'
Nineteenth-century proverb

Kit's words...

For a number of years June Lawson and I made jam to sell in the shop in Brecon, which we ran to raise funds for the Research Trust for Metabolic Diseases in Children. We would use whatever fruit was in season and whatever kind friends were willing to donate from their gardens. Our reputation grew and rhubarb and ginger, plum, damson, raspberry and blackcurrant jams, bottled in recycled jars, were firm favourites with our customers. June also made chutney – then, for days, her kitchen would be filled with heat and the smell of spices as the chutneys simmered in the pan. Green bean chutney – every teaspoon holds a memory now for me.

When we decided that we wanted to buy Upper Albion and establish Harriet's Trust, June was the first to give encouragement: "We've got 22 lbs of blackcurrant jam, it's a start!" and so we began our fund-raising with 22 jars of blackcurrant jam.

At the beginning of July we would look for the 'pick your own strawberries' signs to appear. Then, collecting up our containers and baskets, we would drive to our favourite farm near Hereford. To spend a fine summer morning in a large field in the Herefordshire countryside with the sun, warm on your back, I count as one of life's small but intense pleasures. Finding the sweet-smelling ripe fruit resting on the straw around the plants or under their leaves becomes almost compulsive. The voices of other pickers further away in the field seem to fade and my world shrinks to a sense of warmth, the sweet scarlet fruit aroma mingled with earth and straw. It comes as a regret when the containers are full. I know that the berries are full of ripe flavour from those I have sampled on my journey down the rows. At home a panic of wondering if there are sufficient jars and lemons for juice to help the jam to set before the 'jam-in' begins. Before that, of course, we have to sample the fruit again to make sure that it really is good. After this I don't mind if the rest of the strawberry season passes by without any more bowls of the fruit (served with cream of course) to eat. My greed is well and truly sated.

I can't remember why June and I were sitting on the terrace overlooking her garden, but it was sunny and peaceful in the 'top' village. Llangynidr starts at the old pack-bridge crossing the River Usk, goes up the hill over the Brecon and Monmouth Canal, and finishes further on where the road rises to cross the mountain to Beaufort. We were enjoying a cup of tea and some of June's delicious homemade lemon-drizzle cake. Her phone rang and Grant, one of her neighbours from 'further up' the road, asked if we would like some Victoria plums of which he had more than his family would use. Perhaps from his more elevated position he could see us sitting, idly talking. Ten minutes later he appeared around the corner of the house pushing his wheelbarrow which was overflowing with fruit. We looked at the bounty with a mixture of gratitude and hysteria. A wheelbarrow full of ripe Victoria plums is a wonderful, and an awesome sight. For the dedicated home-based jam maker, a garage containing a large chest freezer is as essential as a preserving pan. Luckily we had both.

Now that John and I have moved to Pembrokeshire, to be closer to the Trust properties, I no longer make so much jam. More occasional coffee mornings and table sales suit my increasing age. The river of jars for recycling that used to flow through our Breconshire home has stopped. However a small spring of jars has welled up in Pembrokeshire. I shall work hard to control the flow.

June Lawson's words...

We made endless amounts of jams and chutneys. I used to ask people in the village for any surplus fruit or vegetables but, one day, I wished I hadn't when a couple arrived on my doorstep with a laundry basket full of runner beans! I happened to have several friends for afternoon tea in the garden, so they were all issued with knives and we spent the rest of the afternoon slicing runner beans prior to making chutney with them. I only acquired a food processor long after we had finished selling chutney. We found a damson tree one day in the garden of a house which was only occupied on rare occasions, so we thought it was a shame to waste the fruit. But we were caught up the ladder, while helping ourselves, by one of the local builders. He didn't report us. Then we spent hours trying to get stones out of the jams as we couldn't risk choking somebody. My other abiding memory is peeling a whole SACK of potatoes for a sausage and mash and jazz evening! We also did several garden open days. I thought my garden was looking quite tidy until a visiting lady said that my garden was her favourite because it had weeds in it just like hers at home!

CHAPTER 19

Musical Moments

'The singing will never be done'
Siegfried Sassoon – 'Everyone Sang', 1916

"DO YOU THINK they'll ever stop singing and go home to bed?" muttered Kit, taking a discreet look at John's wristwatch and fixing the smile more securely on her face, "It's almost half-past eleven," a note of desperation could be heard in her voice. There are night owls and there are early birds and Kit is definitely not one of the nocturnal creatures. After 10 p.m. she becomes less sociable (morose even, say some) as the need to sleep becomes more insistent. It's not that we had never been to a male voice choir concert before, but only as part of the audience when we had thoroughly enjoyed the music and singing and then gone straight home. This time we were responsible for all the arrangements for a concert. Harriet was still managing to find new opportunities and experiences for us.

In our innocence we knew nothing of the after-concert 'concert' that was customary (at least in that part of Wales where we lived) as the choir members and their guests enjoyed light refreshments and wet their collective whistles, preferably at the bar, before the coach came, usually at about 11.45 p.m. That is, if it was a visiting choir. A local choir in our new-found experience might sing a bit longer.

The Abertillery Orpheus Male Choir was one of the first to sing for the Trust. We chose the Manor Hotel at Crickhowell for the venue, set on the hillside overlooking the Usk valley

155

below. The ballroom had been laid out with chairs to seat 300 people. It was a hot evening in early July 1993, and the room was full to capacity. As well as the choir numbers, there were solos from a guest artist, on this occasion a young mezzo-soprano. On that evening there was also to be two recitations from 'The Outing' by Dylan Thomas. The concert was a great success and afterwards the singing continued with equal vigour and volume until the coach arrived to take everyone home. We remember other concerts and other choirs: The Brecon Male Choir, Talgarth Choir; a combined choir concert arranged by a friend who sang with the Brecon Choir and, latterly, Tenby Male Voice Choir has given several concerts for us. Over the 20 years of fund-raising we have heard some wonderful voices lifted in song. In Brecon, one wintry night in the Castle of Brecon hotel (in the same room where Harriet's christening tea was held) we sat and listened to an unaccompanied, impromptu concert after the audience had all gone. One chorister after another singing a favourite hymn or song. 'The Lily of the Valley' is one that lingers in the memory. 'Myfanwy' is another. Beautiful a cappella singing:

> Paham mae dicter, O Myfanwy,~
> Yn llenwi'th lygaid duon di?
> A dweud
> Y gair Ffarwel

No matter that the words were in Welsh and we didn't know all their meaning in English. The poet Shelley understood this perfectly when he wrote:

> Music, when soft voices die,
> Vibrates in the memory.

Certain songs and arrangements are popular with most male choirs. 'The Rhythm of Life' is almost obligatory as is an arrangement of 'The Battle Hymn of the Republic' to bring the concert to an arousing finale. Songs from the musicals, from

Novello through Rogers and Hammerstein to Schönberg (*Les Misérables*) and Lloyd Webber (*Aspects of Love*). Popular songs old and new, folk songs of American, English or Welsh origins, all delivered with enthusiasm to audiences who love to hear their old favourites finely sung.

Over the years those choirs have made not an inconsiderable financial contribution to Harriet's Trust. Among our scrapbook of press cuttings is a rather blurry picture of us posing with the Brecon Choir. The legend reads: "A cheque for £2,506.94 has been presented to John and Kit Davis of the Harriet Davis Trust for Disabled Children by officials of the Aberhonddu and District Male Choir. The money is the proceeds of the successful combined choirs' charity concert held at the Theatr Brycheiniog in September." "I remember that", says John, "Frank Henessey from Radio Wales was the compère for the evening."

In recent times we no longer take such an active part in the arrangements. After concert gatherings and the late-late nights are behind us. Tenby Male Choir give regular concerts for various charitable causes and we are fortunate to take our turn to benefit. Summer visitors to the seaside mingle with local people to fill the pews in the light and airy St Mary's Church in the middle of the town. We sit waiting to present bouquets of flowers to the guest soloist and the accompanist. The conductor, as he always does, invites any holidaying choir member in the audience to come and join in the finale, 'An American Trilogy', and a man who says he is from Cornwall goes down the aisle to take his place amongst the baritones. Through the windows on the south side of the nave we can see the sky getting darker. The choir starts to sing, the rising crescendo of voices fills the church accompanied suddenly by a startling sheet of lightning across the, by now, black summer evening sky. There is a tremendous roll of thunder almost directly overhead the church and the rain pours down. Inside the main lights flicker and die leaving only the Side Chapel lit. Almost imperceptibly at first, the organist joins in the music, the choir sings on, their voices nearly drowning out the sound of the storm. Now the organ thunders as if in unison with the rolls of thunder and flashes of lightning outside. The final Amen rises, the church is filled with sound. As the singing reaches a triumphant end, all the lights come back on and the storm eases. Getting ready to leave, some of the audience think that the lights were dimmed deliberately to add atmosphere. There is no denying that it was a dramatic effect and end to the evening.

At the other end of the scale was the small Girls in Harmony choir from Pontypool who, in August 2002, gave a concert in another favourite venue for choirs – St John's, with its raked pews and gallery. This was where the Jasperian Theatre had performed for us. The Tenby Soroptomist organization had arranged everything for the concert. Brigette Thomas was an ebullient and amusing hostess as she introduced her choir of twelve young women. Such a variety of song: 'Fields of Gold', 'Amazing Grace', 'The Card Song', 'Sleepytime Bach', such a richness of talent amongst them.

And who could forget the Bravo 4? Equally talented, but wholly different in style from the choirs. A well-known barbershop singing group based in Crickhowell, they were pensioners who travelled around Wales and parts of England entertaining folk with their close harmony singing. In December 2003 we went with Anne and Mike Chamberlain (who, you will remember, hedged their bets in Pembrokeshire) to receive a cheque from the quartet – the proceeds from donations given at their performances during that year. As we had not actually heard them sing before, we were treated to an intimate private concert in the upstairs room of that well-known hostelry, The Bear hotel. So we raise our glasses to you: Keith Purkiss, David Handley, Andrew Walker and Stan Walker, who so enjoyed raising your voices in song, for your generosity of heart and time.

Banjos and Bangers is perhaps a phrase to conjure with. The idea must have come from Reg Baynham: mature, quietly spoken, spare in stature but a man of many parts. During World War II he was based at Pembroke Dock working with the Sunderland Flying Boats, and had a fund of interesting stories to tell about his experiences. A talented wood turner, he produced some beautiful small objects for us to sell to help increase Trust funds. He was still an avid cyclist and helped organize a fund-raising bicycle time trial for us. But surely the Banjos and Bangers evening event was his finest hour. The Banjo Band, of which Reg was a member, was anxious to help the Trust and proposed an evening of musical entertainment in Llangynidr's old wooden village hall which had a good stage for the musicians. We decided that Banjos, together with bangers and mash, would offer food for both spirit and body. Calculating how many could be seated to eat in the hall, and the quantities of food needed, we persuaded about 80 friends and supporters to buy tickets.

The kitchen in the old hall was inadequately equipped for our needs and so the food was prepared and cooked at various houses throughout the village and brought to the hall at the last minute. Adele Jones bravely volunteered to prepare onions, and June's experience of peeling a sack of potatoes is still seared upon her memory. On the late autumn evening, steaming hot baked beans and sausages appeared, as if by magic, to be ladled out onto plates with onions and mashed potatoes. A line of kitchen helpers had also appeared, as usual, as if by magic. It is, in our experience, one of the wonders and mysteries of fund-raising: women, who without any fuss, appear and organize the all-important kitchen work. Often, without any specific urging or asking, there they are, preparing food, making tea, washing up and clearing things away.

The six Banjo players were on stage, instruments plugged into an amplifying system. The hall was pleasantly full with the smell of sausages and mash, and the hum of conversation and laughter of the diners. The accompanying musical beat was rhythmical and lively. We began to relax with the satisfied feeling of successful fund-raisers when, abruptly, the hall was plunged into darkness and musical silence. Conversation and laughter also stopped short whilst a torch was found to shed some light upon the electricity meter. One of the kitchen ladies, a regular user of the hall, asked John where the money to feed the meter was. Muttering that no-one had told him he had to provide food for the meter as well as the guests, he began to sort through the 'float-money' tin. "That's no good," said the nameless villager, "that's new money. It's got to be old florins – from the hall secretary. You should have got some beforehand."

The old coin-in-the-slot electricity meter was of such venerable age that it would only accept pre-decimalization coins. As the coinage was changed in 1973, for something over 20 years a supply of old two shilling pieces had been kept to put in the meter at functions taking place in the hall. John put on a fine turn of speed as he hastened to the secretary's house (thankfully fairly nearby) for a supply of coins. Apparently these were later retrieved from the meter to be used over and over again. After the hiatus, light and sound were restored and the evening continued with no more alarms and excursions. Everyone who came voted it a great success in spite of (or perhaps because of) the temporary stoppage. Whenever we hear the lively and rhythmical beat of ukulele or banjo, there we are again, back in the old wooden village hall with Reg and the banjo 'boys' strumming away for Harriet.

CHAPTER 20

Hundreds and Thousands

'There is no new thing under the sun'
Ecclesiastes 1:8

SMALL CHARITIES, LIKE Harriet's Trust, are very reliant upon the goodwill and generosity of many people who give both small and larger amounts of money to help achieve their aims. From the £20 saved as five penny pieces over many months by elderly or very young friends, to the several thousands of pounds from a more adventurous event. Individuals, small groups, schools, service organizations, businesses, banks and building societies, all make their own unique contribution. Often we are asked to talk about the work of the Trust to local groups of these organizations, and have developed a double act of chat and information which we adapt according to the age and number of the listeners. We can follow-up these talks with an invitation to visit one or other of the houses. Orange squash and biscuits for Brownies, Cubs, Scouts and Guides and lively questions about the equipment are as enjoyable as the more sedate but equally interesting times spent chatting over tea and Welsh cakes with groups of those of more mature years. Some of those groups go on to hold an event especially for us, or include Harriet's Trust in the 'end of year' sharing out of their charitable giving. Their tremendous investment of time and effort should never be undervalued. Coffee mornings rarely flop. The cake stall and raffle are always sure-fire money raisers. One group of ladies in Narberth (where Caerwen house is) gave us £600, the proceeds of coffee, biscuits and a raffle, raised in just over an hour. No callow apprentices these, but seasoned fund-raisers with a formidable skill in tapping into their local community. Kit always believes that the amount of money raised at a coffee morning rises exponentially with the decibel level of chat amongst those present.

Just as plants and cuttings for sale are an obligatory part of a 'gardens open' event, so books and bric-a-brac are a fixture at most coffee mornings, table top sales, spring/Christmas/ autumn fairs, car boot sales and garden fêtes – you name it, we've done it.

Bric-a-brac, those myriad small objects, no longer loved, needed or used; teapots and teddies, ornaments of china or glass, gifts given to Granny as a thank you for looking after the dog, cat or garden whilst the family holidayed in Spain or Portugal or Bournemouth. Vases and linens from an elderly relation's house clearance; unwanted bath salts, saucers and saucepans, beads and bangles, hats and handbags, jigsaws and board games, old CDs and videos. The list could stretch to the moon and back. Bric-a-brac and books circulating eternally around the countryside, spilling out from tardis-like homes in any neighbourhood. Do some items, in the manner of raffle – wine for example, barely touch down before being donated on again? We suspect that this is true and that some have been sold many times over, eventually raising more money than their real worth. One thing is for sure, we have never mistakenly (or deliberately) been given a piece of Fabergé jewellery, or Clarice Cliff china, or indeed anything of breath-catching value, to sell on a bric-a-brac stall. A great deal is in good condition and eminently resaleable, but for those things that are not, after ruthless sorting, a final journey to the local amenity tip is inevitable. "No wonder", says John, "that sometimes we feel tired and in need of an afternoon nap!"

An invitation to go to a fund-raising event that we have had no part in organizing or selling tickets for, is always welcome. None of the hard work, none of the worry (will anyone come to support us? Will the weather be reasonable?) but just the pleasure of the event with the bonus of money in the bank for the Trust at the end of it. And thereby hangs another tale: Allotment Antics – or more accurately 'Allotment Anticz'.

Malcolm Melhuish, was one of the first to holiday with his family at Harriet's House in 1994 and now, eighteen years later, not only is still a user but also a Trustee. He phoned to speak to John one day. An idea to raise some funds he said; a calendar featuring the Park Lane allotment holders. The Aberdare, south Wales, Park Lane that is, not the more widely known London one. "No need for you to be involved at all," he told John. "Lovely," we said. "What sort of calendar, how many copies do you think you can sell and for how much?" This is us not being involved. It was October 2009 and we assumed that the calendar would be for the year 2011. Not at all, Malcolm and his fellow allotmenteers intended to complete, print and sell the calendar for 2010 before Christmas. Now we were really worried, only two months? How many copies are you going to print? Where will the set-up money come from and how much will you need? Malcolm was confident of success and we realised that this was no sudden bright idea but a plan that had been unfolding for some time. It had started when a family friend who was moving house offered Malcolm two virtually unused leather settees if the Trust could use them. Harriet's House was in need, and the offer was gratefully accepted. We met Malcolm and two of his fellow allotment holders at the harbour and took delivery of the settees. "Two days later," says Malcolm, "Dave Jenkins, one of the two men who came to Harriet's House phoned. Now I've seen the house, it's really got to my heart. I think the allotment holders should do something to raise some money for your Trust," he exclaimed. After some talking around the subject, Dave and his wife put forward the idea of a calendar. Sweet-talking a local firm in Treforest into giving them thirty large plastic 1,000 litre water holders, they borrowed a flat-bed lorry from another 'mate' and five of them spent one whole day shifting the containers. They sold each water carrier for £12 to other allotment holders in the area – £360 was a good start. Brian Jordan was asked if he would take the photographs without charge. He already knew about Harriet's Trust. As president of Aberdare Lions Club in 1994, he had been involved with their part in funding the first house and had been amongst the many people at the harbour when Harriet's House was officially opened. He agreed to donate his skills with a camera to the cause and, in March 2009, they had 'staged' January, February and December before the background vegetation belied the month date. From then on an idea to represent each month of the unfolding allotment year was set up and the best 'shot' chosen. By the time that Malcolm put the idea to us, it was almost a completed project.

Glynneath Male Voice Choir had agreed to give a concert supporting the allotment holders who could use the money raised to pay for a print run of the calendar. Stevens and George, a local print group, had offered to produce 3,000 calendars. Malcolm, unflappable as ever, said there was plenty of time to do what was needed. They could have the 'goods' ready for sale by the end of the month. The choir concert duly went ahead and raised the hoped for target of £1,000. In a manner reminiscent of the parable of the talents, Malcolm intended to sell the calendars for as little as £3 each, thereby not only covering the printing cost but also doubling his original stake of the proceeds from the concert. He had sponsors and selling outlets arranged in Aberdare market and local shops. We asked to see the calendar and possibly have some to sell as well. Rather grudgingly, Malcolm brought us about two dozen copies, certainly not many more.

It was a calendar to rival that of the famous Calendar Girls. Nine or ten 'old boys' obviously having a good time and enjoying the joke and gentle humour of Allotment Anticz. We can only select one or two to give a flavour of the whole. In March the group watch an allotment game of billiards played with red and white cabbage balls, long-handled broomsticks for cues and a curved-tine hoe as a rest. The mountains in the background look bleak and wintry, and the onlookers, sitting on their plastic allotment chairs, are well wrapped up. Malcolm, pipe in mouth, hat pulled well down against the wind is seated in the middle. 'I'm off the red' reads the caption for the month. Everyone who saw the pictures had their favourite month. One loved the sly humour of September: a summer tanned and fit looking Brian Morris (then responsible for the whole allotment site) wearing only a necktie and a broad smile, posed with a trug full of rhubarb and holding one large leaf to maintain his modesty, 'Rhubarb Fool' – lovely. Another's favourite was the wonderful green face of Dave-the-post (time honoured Welsh custom of name reflecting occupation) peeping out between the row of blooming runner beans. The red flowers and green leaves of the plants giving cover and camouflage to the 'Human Bean' in their midst. His green gardening sunhat and mouth coloured to match the red blooms helping the illusion. Hiding also in the plants is the grinning stone-man face belonging to Malcolm which featured somewhere in each month's picture. We especially like the portrait of Mr Gummidge, chosen for May month when, of course, seedlings are beginning to grow in the early summer sunshine (at least in theory). Those of us old enough to remember the children's stories about Worzel Gummidge, the scarecrow, were delighted to see the re-creation of Barbara Euphan Todd's character. Alfie Crumm, arms outstretched, surveying the world with a slightly 'melancholy' air through the stalks of straw coming down from his hat with more stuffed into his jacket. The stone man this time is nestled against Mr Gummidge's neck, balancing on one outstretched scarecrow-like arm; in some strange way it seems to reflect the wistful look on Alfie's face.

We need not have had any doubts that six weeks was too short a time in which to sell 3,000 calendars. Within two weeks they were sold out, giving us a master class in salesmanship and generosity.

There is in this early part of the twenty-first century, a fashion for big challenges organized by big charities – walking or cycling through areas of extreme climate, 'celebrity' involvement in scaling mountains perhaps, setting tasks which challenge individual personal limits of physical or emotional endurance for which those taking part seek large sums of sponsorship money. Similar challenges are offered and accepted by many non-celebrities too. Things that those of us who are barely fit enough to hasten to catch the approaching bus to town, can never hope to emulate.

One of the better known of these physical challenges takes place every year – the Flora London Marathon – when thousands of ordinary people can apply to compete and raise money for their chosen charity. Over the years we have sat and watched on the television the mass of people starting off from Blackheath. We have followed the day's events and looked closely to see if we could spot 'our' runners, but have never managed to do so. However we do have a permanent official record from the year 2000 marathon. Kevin Griffiths (son of Ruth who looked after Harriet's House), runner number 7,988 pinned to his vest, was photographed running past the Tower of London, with Tower Bridge in the background. He looks relaxed and is running so easily that he is able to look towards the cameraman, smiling all the while. He was obviously going to improve on his previous running time of two hours and forty-seven minutes. John McFall was an earlier and equally doughty runner for the Trust. He and his fellow runners were entertained to dinner by Harriet's uncle and aunt, Paul and Tina, at The George Inn in Southwark which they were managing at that time.

If running 26 miles seems too extreme and not for you, how about trying the madness of the Tenby Boxing Day swim? In its own way no less a physical challenge, but one of shorter duration. On that day every year hundreds of people make their way towards the harbour and adjacent North Beach. As they assemble on the beach, hundreds more line the walkways overlooking it to watch the spectacle. A large, warming, bonfire is ready, the lifeboat on standby, swimmers begin to shrug off outer layers of clothing to reveal all manner of swimwear and fancy dress. Which will be worse? To go into the water dressed only in a skimpy swimming costume or, with less flesh bared, in a costume that will hold the winter-cold water and cling around your body afterwards? Father Christmases, elves, plum puddings, pop star lookalikes, costumes and caricatures of events and people in the news are all there. Each year the organizers set a different theme, with prizes awarded for those judged the best. There is ample opportunity for ingenuity and examples of the Great British carnival humour to be displayed and appreciated. The klaxon sounds out and the colourful human wave flows down the sand to the water's edge. The air is filled with yells of encouragement from the onlookers and screams of excitement, anticipation and shock from the 'dippers'. It is a matter of honour to get wet from head to foot and many do actually swim rather than just cavort about at waist depth. Hot soup and medals are given out close by the warmth of the bonfire. People begin to drift away to warm up in cafés and cars. Before long everyone is gone and the beach is quiet as the incoming tide reclaims its own. The amounts of money raised for the Trust are impressive: ranging from several hundred to more than a £1,000 in various years, our thanks go to families staying in Harriet's House for Christmas, Malcolm, his son Dean and Basil (known to everyone who stays at the Wheelabout) staying either with friends from the local hostelry or on his own. In fact he confessed that it was in the Cross Inn at the end of a merry evening that he was persuaded to take part in his first winter swim. Dark glasses and a hat brought back from a Turkish holiday gave Basil a rather mysterious, louche appearance on the day, but couldn't make the temperature, in or out of the water, anything other than breezily cold.

It is not necessary to actually enter the sea to set a personal challenge or target. You can walk the length of the Pembrokeshire Coastal Path with the sea by your side for 180 miles. James Masterman, who we had never met or knew sent an e-mail in the spring of 2010. He intended to walk the length of the Pembrokeshire Coastal Path in seven days, on his own.

He wanted to raise some money for a locally-based charity and Harriet's Trust was his choice. Over the next few months we met him and approved his plans. He had found bed and breakfast for each night of his journey, without charge. On the day appointed, carrying all he needed for his journey in his rucksack (though without his mobile phone charger as we later discovered), we waved James goodbye at Poppit sands. "Which way is it?" he asked, rather worryingly, as he looked for the acorn sign on the signpost. "Keep following the acorn and the sea to your right hand," we called after him. We watched his progress up the lane to the cliff path. "I hope he'll be alright," we said to each other. "He's set himself a very hard goal." On the third day, because his phone needed recharging, we heard nothing until the evening when he reached his stopover. He assured us that all was well and he was enjoying meeting many people on his way who showed him much kindness. His longest stretch of the walk was to end at Stackpole Quay and his overnight stay was at the Stackpole Arms in the village. It began to get dark, nearly 9 p.m., and still no sign or phone call. Who to call first? Perhaps he had fallen and injured himself, or worse still, fallen down the cliffs into the sea and drowned. Coastguard, Lifeboat, we fretted? We were greatly relieved when the phone rang to say that he had arrived safely. A big cheer greeted him as he entered the bar and a meal was put before him before he fell asleep. At the end of the seven days he admitted that an old injury to his ankle had made the walk, "one of the hardest things I've ever done." The £1,000 raised helped sweeten his pain and we, of course, were grateful for his generous support. The kindness of strangers is a never ending surprise to us, and so many who start as strangers, end as friends.

Another long-distance event happened early on when Harriet's House, on the harbour at Tenby, was our only property. Marathon cyclists John Kaffenberger and Mark Sieven rode from Guildford to Tenby. They were seen off by James and Sue Molyneux at Loseley Park on a Friday morning and arrived in Tenby later in the weekend to be met by David Manby and us. The Kaffenberger family, who then lived in Croydon, was among the first to use Harriet's House. Their son, Andrew, was wheelchair dependent and we really appreciated the fact that they found time to support our work, in spite of all the difficulties in their own lives.

Fund-raising events are only, then, restricted by the limits of one's imagination and considerations of safe practice. We have never been particularly adventurous or, we think, particularly good at fund-raising events, but we have had some great fun over the years that we have been responsible for instigating or organizing.

An evening that we particularly enjoyed happened in 2009. Mark Drewitt of Carrington's Restaurant in Tenby, a favourite eating place of ours for several years, wanted to host a dinner for the Trust. We invited 40 guests, sufficient to fill the intimate dining room, and asked an old friend, Roy Noble, if he would provide the after dinner speech. Without cost to us, Mark, his suppliers and his young chef Phillip, provided, planned and prepared a high-class five-course meal. Our only contribution was the payment for the young waitresses. All the rest was profit for the Trust. We were delighted with the enthusiastic replies of all who were invited. Roy Noble had been one of the very first people to see Harriet after she was born, as he was then headmaster of a junior school and was a colleague of John's at work. He subsequently became a very well-known and loved presenter on Radio Wales. A raconteur in the finest Welsh tradition, after an excellent meal, he kept all the guests convulsed in gales of laughter as he reminisced about life in Wales.

If we have learnt anything from our fund-raising activities, it is that there is little new and little that hasn't already been done somewhere else. We also have learnt not to take personally a refusal to participate or buy a ticket for something. There are scores of charitable causes, from large international or national to local small charitable ones, all deserving of support and people choose which one they will. Most importantly, though, we must never forget to say thank you. From the elderly gentleman who makes a modest annual contribution, to the large grant-making trust, each deserves a thank you. Whenever we have sought and been given financial support from grant-making trusts, John has always followed the same routine: a) write and say thank you and b) later on write again to say how the money has been spent, to underline our thanks. Once, having been given a grant of £5,000 and done both steps a) and b), he was surprised to receive another cheque for the same amount. Perplexed, he phoned the grant administrator because he thought they had mistakenly sent more. But no, "We very rarely get a thank you or to know that the money has actually been spent properly," was the reply. "We thought we would like to give you some more to show how much we appreciated your letters."

We were almost as surprised by that as we have been by the willingness of others to put a hand in their pocket or purse and spend their money to help us achieve our modest aims. All we can do is to thank all the hundreds of people who have shown such generosity with time or money or love and make sure that we do not thoughtlessly squander any of these gifts.

CHAPTER 21

Hold the Fort

'Hold the fort for I am coming.'

P P Bliss – 'Ho my Comrades'

IT WOULD HAVE been in April 2005 when the young woman at the Big Lottery Fund office was quick to remind us of Kit's words last time we had met in late April 2002: "If I ever, ever, get in touch to say we want a grant to do another house – just shoot me." "Would you like me to bring the gun with me?" she asked. She wanted to know what had happened in the three years since completing the Wheelabout project to bring about such a volte-face. Very simply, the number of enquiries from families of children with learning disabilities or who were autistic was increasing year on year. Whilst some had additional physical disabilities which made the special equipment in the houses a necessity for their proper care, others were not wheelchair dependent which was a problem for us. In theory those who were not in need of the equipment for their physical care, could find holiday accommodation in any one of the hundreds of self-catering cottages and apartments easily found through the annual publications of commercial firms. In reality, their needs could be just as special and difficult to satisfy as those arising from physical disabilities. In 2002, we had opened a small office in Tenby, run on a part-time basis by Helen Lees-Griffiths who had looked after Harriet's House for some years after Ruth Griffiths retired. Helen, who was now dealing with all the bookings for the houses, was also concerned about the growing number of enquiries from families whose needs were not being met.

Our knowledge and experience of autism was limited and largely academic. What we did learn from that limited experience was that all three of our houses, which had been designed to cope with wheelchairs, contained a lot of expensive equipment which could be vulnerable to damage. Once, for example, the lift button in Giltar View was pressed so many times that eventually it refused to function. Perseverance is quite a common behaviour trait in autistic children, when the same movement is repeated over and over. Several door handles were broken in this way. On another occasion the 'Henry' vacuum cleaner was taken out of its cupboard and dismantled by one small boy. The repairman was quite impressed, "he almost got the motor re-assembled correctly," he said (but not sufficiently for it to work). After the washing machine had been used as a cement mixer, with copious amounts of sand put into it, we decided that we would either have to refuse to take any bookings from autistic children or offer something more suited to their needs.

We consulted the National Autistic Society to learn more about the disability. We found their document about autism in relation to building design to be succinct and clear.

It describes autism as a lifelong condition, characterised by three main features: impairment of social relationships; impairment of communication skills; impairment of imagination.

These could lead to a display of behaviour which could have an impact on buildings: that is obsessional behaviour, hyperactive behaviour and behavioral tantrums. 'A high proportion of those with autism have associated learning difficulties and may also suffer from epilepsy' (taken from the National Autistic Society's architects' briefing notes).

We continued our consultations by talking to the Welsh branch of the National Autistic Society and with parents of autistic children and carers groups. We also visited a newly-opened respite unit for children with autism in Brecon and saw for ourselves some of its special design features and equipment. The staff there was helpful and gave us sensible advice. Gradually we arrived at the point of resolving to provide a holiday house especially for autistic children. John asked the same question of everyone he talked to: "Will there be enough need for a dedicated property to make it economically viable?" The answer was always unequivocal: "I could fill it from my case-load alone" (a social worker from south-east Wales); "I think they'd bite your hand off" (a worker at the Autistic Society); "Yes please. Of course it is needed. It would be well used" (a parent). We were convinced, and that is how we came to be talking to the young woman at the Big Lottery Fund office in the spring of 2005. Another major grant from their funds would enable us to buy a suitable property to adapt.

Off we went for the third time. John was becoming ever more skilled with computer technology, even if his sighs of despair as he sat in front of the computer screen made it seem otherwise. This time he downloaded the forms and completed them on the computer before printing them. We felt childishly pleased with this accomplishment. The forms were little changed since our first application nine years previously. Questions about who would benefit, how the project would achieve our aims and what changes it would bring about for those it benefited were liberally peppered with words like 'outcomes' and 'outputs' and rather convoluted phrases such as: "How will you know if the outputs are helping your beneficiaries achieve the outcomes identified in B1?" But we were seasoned form fillers and our project was, in essence, quite simple to describe. As before, detailed budgets and business plans were asked for. This information was readily to hand from John's discussions with the other Trustees and from the Trust accounts. We intended to ask for £245,000 towards the purchase of the property and find the rest of the costs from our own resources and fund-raising efforts. We had come a long way since 1996 and the large sums of money involved no longer frightened us.

The time between sending our application in late May and the September meeting of the Lottery grants committee when we expected a decision to be made, was very busy for us. We were making our plans to move to Tenby by Christmas of that year and, although we looked forward to going, we had been in the house in Llangynidr for more than 20 years and in Breconshire for nearly 30. We knew that we would miss our many friends there but, by now, we had formed friendships in Pembrokeshire as well. It was not as if we were going somewhere entirely unknown.

In due course we were delighted to learn that our application was successful. We said our farewells to Brecon and the house in Llangynidr with all their memories, both sad and happy. In Pembrokeshire we began the by now familiar search for a house for Harriet's Trust. Twenty houses were looked at and rejected. Too small, too big, unsuitable layout, too close to its neighbours, too isolated, too far from the beaches. Houses number 21, 22, 23 – still nothing suitable. We began to despair and worry a little about the time limits for completing the project. We saw an advert for a house that might fit our wish list: not isolated, with a level back garden that could be made secure, no close neighbours, big enough for our purpose and, most importantly, within our proposed budget. The 28th house we had viewed. Hurrah! We needed to look no further. From the house it is an easy walk into the little market town of Narberth where there is a good selection of independent shops, and places to eat. The beaches of Amroth, Wiseman's Bridge and Saundersfoot are all close by.

It felt strange not to have to make major alterations inside the house. Everything was in good condition and the rooms were spacious and light. The most important changes involved preparing one of the two large sitting rooms to be a soft play room. The old gas fire and back boiler needed removing and the gas supply to the house, which came into this room, had to be re-routed. The electric sockets in the room were covered and the light switch on the wall changed. The advice we had been given was that plastic fittings for switches and power sockets should be avoided. Brass and anodised aluminium were less easily damaged. The low window overlooking the front garden in the soon-to-be soft play room was replaced with one that would allow the wall cushions to be properly fixed. The light fittings throughout the house were changed so that there were no hanging flexes; we had also learnt that light fittings, door handles and window catches should be of a consistent design throughout.

We did our best to carry out all the safety advice we had been given. George Gunnell, a master carpenter before becoming principal carer to Ben, came for a week while Ben was in respite care. George, with his wife Gwen acting as carpenter's 'boy', fitted 'starlocks' to all the room doors and childproof locks to all the kitchen cupboards. This was a tedious and time consuming task, and we appreciated their generous gift of time and expertise.

We had been given a grant from a Charitable Trust to pay for the installation of the soft playroom. A young woman from 'Rompa', a firm specialising in soft play and sensory rooms, came to measure for the made-to-measure floor and wall cushions. We had looked carefully at the catalogue of play equipment and made our choice: several collections of different sized soft shapes which could be used for imaginative play. One phrase that we had heard many times was 'low stimulus environment' – no busy patterns, but calming colours where possible. Florinda Toms, now one of the Trustees, and Kit studied the catalogue and colour samples at length. Perhaps the caramel colour for the wall and floor cushions? The young woman from Rompa looked a little doubtful. "Oh blow it" said Kit, "it would look too boring and sickly". Orange floor and yellow walls; a deep purple wave shape for rolling down; green, blue and yellow shapes for building blocks – one set called liquorice allsorts looks exactly like the sweets in colour and shape. The finished room positively vibrates with colour. What is more, none of the families have complained about the bright scheme.

Elsewhere we did observe the low stimulus advice. Muted plain colours, for walls and floor covering, toned with plain curtaining material. We had been told that curtains would be an easy target for hyperactive behaviour and temper tantrums. But, to provide the electronically controlled blinds between doubled glazed units that we had seen, was out of our reach financially. We compromised with lightweight fittings and easy fixtures, so that as little damage as possible could happen to either house or human.

Once again the Probation Service provided the labour force to decorate inside and help with the outside work. One of the most expensive and difficult jobs outside was to put six-foot high fencing all round. The young man, Dean, who came to do it, worked long hours digging and fixing. The worst bit he said was having to get behind the leylandii hedge (about eight-foot high) to secure the boundaries between us and our next door neighbour – the police station (never any trouble from them anyway). On the other side of the garden the fence created a useful neutral space before the original field hedge of trees. Here the garden shed, bins for compost and rubbish and other necessities would be safe from interference. There were daffodils, snowdrops, violets, celandines and ferns at the base of the old trees of ash, sycamore and hawthorn. Because the fencing is not boarded, but of a paling design, the flowers and green shade still seem to be part of the overall garden. The probation 'boys' dug out several old shrubs in the back garden. There we have now created a raised bed full of culinary herbs which, if leaves are chewed, will not cause any great digestive problems, even if the taste is not very pleasant.

The house name on the front entrance gate is 'Caerwen'. In Welsh the word 'Caer' means a fortified enclosure or fortress and 'wen' can mean white, fair or pleasant. We hope that our Caerwen is indeed a pleasant, safe enclosure for the families. As with the Wheelabout and Giltar View, we did not change the original name of the house. It was not until afterwards that we all appreciated its aptness. A new junior school for Narberth has recently been built on the fields on the other side of Caerwen, but it has not made any difference to our holidaymakers. We had a visit from a delegation of the children who gave their harvest collection for us to use. We put the money towards an original work of art, something we have done in each house.

At Caerwen all the pictures are framed behind Perspex and screwed firmly to the wall. The furniture is heavy and, as far as possible, without sharp edges. Chris Hughes of T P Hughes in Tenby asked if he could put us forward to be chosen as charity of the year by Halo Furniture, one of his suppliers. We had already decided to buy a large dining table and chairs from Halo for Caerwen. We had seen it in Chris's shop. "It's exactly right," said Kit. "No sharp edges, and so heavy it's almost immovable." We were delighted to be chosen as winner and were invited to choose some furniture as our prize. Not being sure how much to ask for, we wrote out a wish list of the dining table with six chairs, two book cases, a double bed and a wardrobe, thinking that the firm could then decide how much to give. To our surprise we were given everything on our wish list. The prize was worth nearly £5,000 to the Trust in saved expenditure. Such a sum is rarely given as a small grant which normally is in the hundreds, not thousands, of pounds. As always it is often the unexpected gift which touches deeply.

When the dozen children from the newly-built school came to visit with their harvest service donation, they gave the soft playroom a test run. Gathered in the sitting room at the beginning of their visit they were shyly quiet and polite. Then came the invitation to take off their shoes and go into the playroom. Almost immediately the house resounded with laughter and talk. We knew then that we had made the right choices for the room. More recently we received another unexpected gift of money in a legacy from an elderly lady who in fact we did not remember meeting, but who obviously knew about Harriet's Trust. We spent some of the money on the back garden. An area of ugly old and cracked concrete outside the back door has been transformed into a soft play area. The surface is now sky-blue rubberised material of the type often used by local authorities in children's play areas and school playgrounds. Set into the sky-blue background is a vivid hop-scotch pattern with squares and numbers in orange, yellow and green. This time Kit wasn't afraid to go for bright colours. Six or seven children on their way home from school came to look and, without commenting, immediately hopped and jumped up the grid of squares and then voted it a success.

The official opening, in early May 2007, was a family affair with Bishop Dewi Bridges once again blessing the project in the company of all the Trustees. We had all brought contributions for a buffet-style lunch and were content to just sit and relax in a little glow of achievement. Caerwen had been the most trouble free of our projects to get ready and we hoped that this augured well for its future. Friends, old and new, came to visit on open day, 27 May 2007. Their comments were all complimentary, but naturally the real test of success would be if the families coming to holiday at Caerwen, our 'fair and pleasant' fortress, were equally complimentary – and they have been.

CHAPTER 22

Field Days with Kit

'Thistle and darnel and dock grew there,
And a bush, in the corner of May'
Walter de la Mare (1873–1956) – 'Nicholas Nye'

WHEN THE LAND at the Wheelabout was bought by Harriet's Trust, the field next to the old cottage and garden looked sad and neglected: not just 'set aside' land but more like forgotten about. The pasture was rough with a mixture of tough grasses such as darnel (a type of rye), dock and thistle that would have gladdened the heart of any donkey, let alone the one celebrated by Walter de la Mare. In the overgrown hedge, half-buried in bramble and stinging nettles, were an old bath full of stagnant water, obviously once used as a drinking trough for animals, old rusting farm implements and a broken wheelbarrow. But it was love at first sight. I barely noticed the hideous phone mast in the top corner of the little three-quarter of an acre meadow. The land sloped down towards the road. The field gate led into the narrow quiet Strawberry Lane and, from this top end of the field, the view looks towards the Preseli Hills in one direction, and towards Tenby town and the sea in the other. This was my field and I loved it. The fact that it wasn't really mine was no matter.

The damage done to the little field during the building works was disheartening and I found it hard to believe that the rubble and debris would ever be cleared properly or that the land would recover from the sea of mud created by heavy machinery and winter gales. Before the construction workers left they did at least level the ground after burying some of the rubble along the top edge of the field. On the Strawberry Lane side the part of the old hedge bank which had been destroyed was rebuilt ready for replacement hawthorn and blackthorn plants. A small wooden gate gave easy access to the field from the garden. New fencing between the little gate and the bank above Holloway Lane defined the garden boundary and later we planted a hedge of hardy fuchsia along its length.

Within a year the land had reverted to a waist high mixture of grasses, clovers, thistle, ragwort and dock. My ambition was to turn this into a wildflower meadow; fuelled no doubt by a visit to Prince Charles' garden at Highgrove and seeing the lovely wildflower meadow there. Life, alas, is full of compromise if not disappointment of ambition. It quickly became obvious that we had neither the physical strength nor the time to achieve a wild flower meadow. Top soil would have had to be removed; the area was too small to be cut with farm machinery, we were not strong enough to use strimmers (the noisy but effective form of the old-fashioned scythes) to cut the long grass. Raking the grass by hand when cut would be a mammoth task. The financial resources of the Trust were very limited and the field a low priority.

I accepted the reality of what we might achieve – over a period of years, by cutting and raking in a patchwork fashion, perennial wildflowers could be encouraged to return; by removing some of the thistle and dock each year there would not be as much competition for the less vigorous plants to contend with. We also wanted to make parts of the field wheelchair friendly. There was plenty of challenge in my modified ambitions.

The probation boys were called in to help. Sunday morning hush would be broken by seven or eight harsh, strident, strimmers sounding like a swarm of angry monster bees as the group cut through the long grass. Raking up the cuttings afterwards was hard work and some of the young men were noticeably less enthusiastic as they bent to the task. It was always the Sunday group who helped us. They were those offenders who had full-time jobs and so had to fulfill their community work obligations on Sundays. They had all been told about the purpose of the Trust and generally worked hard. We always told them how much we appreciated their contribution.

I wanted to create some paths which would wind through the long grasses and flowers – green grassy paths that were firm, smooth and wide enough for a wheelchair. John retreated into his office and, as ever, after making various phone calls to a number of contacts, emerged with the solution: plastic sturdy netting laid on a bed of sand and hogging (that sounded interesting) and then the grass allowed to establish over what would be a firm foundation. This was the basic system used in some rural public car parks where tarmac would be unacceptable. We would not need the heaviest gauge of mesh as cars would not be using the paths. Steve Laughton, the probation group's supervisor, made light of the task. He advised John how much sand and hogging (a sort of coarse grit/dust) to order and a huge roll of plastic netting was delivered together with dumper bags of hogging.

Before this, on a cool and blustery day, after the grass had been cut and raked, a motley crew gathered in the field. The McFall family (they never did learn to say no), the Melhuish family with Laura in her wheelchair, and John and me. Margaret Melhuish manfully pushed Laura around the bumpy ground whilst the rest of us debated the best layout for the paths. Then Malcolm and John marked the route with yellow spray paint. Laura did not seem to mind the shaking of lungs, teeth and head as her wheelchair lurched about the ground.

The paths were laid and gradually the field took shape.

Jenny Axon and her young worker, David, began to take on the bulk of the field work with my help (or interference) when possible. Ad hoc raking parties would be got together when the long grass cut was finished. New friends and old are still persuaded to bring a rake to the field and enjoy a happy morning in the timeless activity of handraking the mown grass.

The 'boy David' had my top two essential requirements in a gardening assistant, strong knees and wrists. He often arrived late in his battered old car with numerous tales of personal or domestic drama. A pink fuzzy hat of uncertain provenance was his favoured head-covering, although occasionally his hair would be dyed green and given an airing. He was always short of cash and sometimes brought an equally hapless mate with him. He was an entertaining and good-natured worker – Jenny had taught him well. He worked steadily and hard at whatever tasks he was given. When Jenny did less work in the field, David was quite capable of taking over. Every year he, his family and Jenny would journey to Glastonbury to the music festival. "I'm going to Glastonbury on Friday. I'll see you the week after next. I'll need a few days to recover," said David. He disappeared down the lane in his old car and has never since reappeared in the field. Better offers of work came his way and quite rightly he took them up. I still have news of him via Jenny and he has earned his place in the story of the taming of the field.

We have invested a large amount of money in a wheeled strimmer specially designed to tackle long grass on rough ground. Basil, who looks after the house and grounds, has become quite attached to the monster 'Grillo' and the field has, at last, after nine years of work, fulfilled my more modest ambitions. A wooden bench placed at the top of the field looks towards the Preseli Hills. Jo and Basil built and decorated a seat within a trellised alcove just inside the small gate from the garden. Seashells, mirrored shapes and pieces of old blue and white china embellish the plinth and the seat, an appropriated (with full owners' consent, once they knew its intended new life) large slab of beautiful old Welsh slate is cool to rest on in the shade of the hedge. The grassy paths are established and during the growing season Basil keeps them mown short. He has also established a wider swathe of closely mown grass stretching down the sloping area of the meadow towards the apple trees.

One of our neighbours in Llangynidr was an elderly man, Eric Brown, who had been a forester during his working life. After Harriet's death and Eric grew frailer, I would visit him for a cup of tea and chat. In spite of his failing limbs and eyesight, his mind was clear and active. We talked about many things but especially about gardening and the countryside. He kindled in me a renewed interest in trees and he had a deep knowledge of many British native species. In the very centre of the little field at the Wheelabout is a hawthorn tree – *Laciniata* – in memory of Eric and his wife Nancy. Around the little tree amongst the grasses I have introduced some Tenby daffodils (the original wild narcissus of Pembrokeshire) and blue camassia, small spikes of intense spring colour which are multiplying rapidly. Light blue field scabious, oxeye daisies, creamy plumes of meadow sweet and the pink of field mallow and fluffy hemp agrimony follow in their season. There are bluebells and red campion in the hedgerows. Altogether over 30 varieties of wildflower can now be found amongst the hedges and grasses.

About the field we have planted 15 trees, each one for a child who we have known from their holidays with Harriet's Trust. These are some of the children who, like Harriet, have been unable to keep hold of their fragile link to life, but who live on in the memory of their families and friends. Bishop Dewi Bridges, now retired back to Tenby, helped Jo and I to plant narcissi around each tree and in places about the field where we hope they will naturalise well. The field has been rechristened as Star Meadow reflecting perhaps the traditional American Indian Folk Tale about the stars. In the 'Song of Hiawatha' the poet Longfellow writes:

> Many things Nokomis taught him
> Of the stars that shine in heaven...
> showed the broad white road in heaven;
> Pathway of the ghosts, the shadows,
> Running straight across the heavens,
> Crowded with the ghosts, the shadows.

On a calm day, Star Meadow has become a peaceful place to sit and reflect upon many things. At other times it is a good place to run and play or be pushed around the little grassy paths and watch the varied flowers, plants and insects that now flourish there.

The monster in the corner has proved to be immoveable. I do not dwell upon the modern inexorable march of the mobile phone masts; as an unrepentant Luddite it does my blood pressure no good to do so. In our meadow the ugly wire fencing with barbed wire along the top enclosing the mast has been hidden behind an outer wooden paling fence. Holly bushes screen it further and a little group of conifers are growing apace to obscure the mast from the house and garden. It's another compromise I've had to make and the annual rental paid to the Trust is put to good use. The service engineers have learnt to tread softly and when site visits are needed, observe the protocols (lovely modern jargon) of good manners. It is good to know that my reputation as a formidable woman remains intact. I have learnt to sit with my back to the enclosure and appreciate the view across the field to the Preselli Hills.

In late May and early June the light sweet scent of a musk rose pervades the air in the field and around the field gate into Strawberry Lane. When we were on holiday in Tenby with Harriet we visited Picton Castle, where she enjoyed driving her wheelchair along the garden paths. There I bought a small cutting of a Paul's Himalayan musk rose which was in full bloom against one of the old walls. "You're mad" exclaimed my sister, "where are you going to put it in your small garden? You do know it will reach 30 feet and more?" "Don't you worry, I'll stuff it in somewhere," I replied. The next morning, Joan and her husband Arthur disappeared for some hours. They returned with not one but two cuttings of the same rose. I said nothing. Just smiled smugly. I knew she would be unable to resist. It has taken eight years for the cutting I brought from Llangynidr to establish itself in the old hedgerow between the meadow and the garden, spreading along the entire length; it is one of the early summer glories of Star Meadow.

Families staying at the house can watch the wildlife in the field. Foxes and their cubs, and tracks of other visitors can be found criss-crossing the grass. Families of toads hide in the damp hedges and butterflies and bees and other small insects work busily. Amongst the birds I can sometimes watch buzzards riding the thermal waves high above the field and listen to their mewling cries. Harriet, as I think I have already written, found gardening 'boring', but I like to think that she would have enjoyed taking her wheelchair around the green pathways, especially if she had some lively company with her.

Interlude
Nearly the Last Word from Angela
– as usual

The Harriet Davis Activity Breaks

Now these are hidden gems of the Trust. Not many know of them but those who have been invited will never forget them. They are a marvellous, exciting sideline for the chosen few.

Activity breaks may be the one-day special, the short break or the de luxe week-long model. The location of such breaks is Tenby, the beautiful seaside location that is enjoyed by thousands of tourists each year and truly blessed by our Harriet Davis families. However, those on the activity breaks are on a hope and a long promise of walks on the beach, sunbathing and relaxation.

If one should be invited on such an excursion pack accordingly – old clothes, suitable footwear – flip-flops, wellies, boots – anything and everything. You could try, with an element of optimism, to pack the book you have saved for holiday reading or the fishing kit, but there is no promise that they will be even seen, let alone used!

Yes – the activity holiday break is always a working holiday. The McFall family has tried out all variations of this unique special offer.

The one-day version; a typical one was moving into house number two, Giltar View. On the way to Tenby, David and Gethyn were treated to breakfast with a beach view in Amroth. A beautiful day and the last they saw of the sea for the next twelve hours. The initial knock on the front door was greeted with Kit yanking open the door. Did we get the usual, "The McFalls, how lovely to see you"? Heck no! It was, "Come in, how good are you with a paint brush? I think I've overdone the yellow paint in the special bedroom!"

While John D, John McFall, David and Gethyn wisely beat a hasty retreat to the kitchen, Angela accompanied Kit upstairs. The brightness of the walls was discussed and it was finally agreed that the sunshine yellow would be toned down once the sheer curtains were hung. Thankfully an hour later this worked.

The day then progressed to carrying anything and everything small that was being delivered by truck or campervan. More friends on the Tenby day-out promise went through the doors of Giltar View that day. Everything was done not only with placement instructions but "mind the wallpaper" – not always easy in a three-storey house and wardrobes etc., have to go around corners and upstairs at the same time. By the time a lunch, tea or was it supper of fish and chips was delivered, we had all had enough activity for one day and the tide had beaten us to the beach. However, a lot had been accomplished.

David even sweet-talked his girlfriend, Nikki, into a day in Tenby. The writing was on the wall when she too was treated to breakfast in Amroth – eaten outside in the early morning sunshine with the sea lapping against the nearby pebbles on the shore. Little did she know then that "Tenby and the sea" would be in the form of a panoramic view from the newest Harriet Davis Trust project – The Wheelabout on the Ridgeway in Penally! That day had a gardening theme – yes clearing out the rubble left by the builders in what was to be the flower and shrub beds. We managed to wear out two buckets and the front wheel of the wheelbarrow commandeered from the builders yard at the end of the site on that occasion. Nikki must have enjoyed herself though – David and Nikki are still together, now joined by their daughter Carys, but still wary of an offer of a day out in Tenby!

Eventually Angela and John progressed through to the de luxe model of Tenby visits. This was an invite for a week's stay at the Wheelabout. Yes! All properties at this time were up and running, gardens planted etc. The invite was on the basis of a break for Angela during a challenging hectic teaching period. The Wheelabout was unoccupied by families and the time could be used for a little maintenance.

At the same time the Melhuish family, Malcolm, Margaret and Laura, would be there. This sounded great. The Melhuish family had become great friends. They had begun as a Harriet Davis holiday family due to Laura needing special accommodation. Then they too had become victims of the magnetic pull of the Trust and that inability to say no to the Davis management. Malcolm had contributed his fantastic skills of being able to paint, paper and fix anything many times. Malcolm had plans for the week.

What finally transpired was the activity holiday to beat all – along with hysterical laughter, good company, meeting and developing a lifelong friendship with Jenny the gardener. Oh, and also backache, cuts, bruises, hypothermia etc. Mind you we were well fuelled by Margaret and Laura's skill in the kitchen. That's one area no-one else is allowed into when they are around, and we bless them for it.

The first morning John D was already at his devious best. "Good morning, lovely day. What do you have planned for the day?" Mm – did he want something? Eventually he just innocently slipped in, "Only I was thinking, if you are thinking of going anywhere today the weather forecast says it will improve later. So if you go into Tenby early you could perhaps do some painting when you come back… if you want to of course!"

Mr D never barks orders, but we always obey. We went in to town, got the paper, said a quick hello to the sea and returned to base. And so the week took shape.

Kit and Jenny in the garden; Malcolm, John and Angela McFall painting and John Davis supervising and doing this and that and anything that needed something technical. The sun did shine, but the wind blew and it was freezing! The back door was finally painted by Angela wearing two T-shirts, a jumper and, by now a ruined, fleece hoody and woolly gloves.

Then came the 'tower scaffold event'. An episode that will be forever remembered by the motley crew. Also formally recognised later at the annual Trustees meeting when Mr D was presented with the framed, tower scaffold health and safety instructions. The external painting project had come to the stage of painting the upstairs windows. Malcolm had convinced John D that a mobile tower scaffold could be hired for the job. Poor John – of all the things he had done for the Trust, this took a toll on his nerves.

When Angela got up at 7.30 a.m., she found Mr D in the kitchen – pacing. Still in his pyjamas and dressing gown he was pacing. He was also holding a sheet of paper. There was a brief exchange of good morning but more importantly what did Angela think the force of the wind outside was on the Beaufort scale? What? Apparently the instructions sheet included health and safety information that the tower was not to be used in certain wind conditions. Sticking your head outside the back door and saying "Cor, it's a bit breezy" didn't count. After breakfast however it was agreed that the task could go ahead. By this time it was a general consensus of the gang that it was a good idea to keep Mr Davis busy – anywhere with anything, as long as it was not near the tower scaffold. Let Malcolm and John McFall get on with it.

Angela still had bits and pieces of window frame and fencing to paint. Jenny was still hard at it in the garden being supervised by Kit – Jenny being the only one who could keep up with Kit's bottomless pit of knowledge of Latin names for flowers. Margaret and Laura would keep us well fed.

All went well until John D escaped all other plans and decided to check on the tower scaffold. This was by now being erected and put into position in the narrow pathway just along from the front door. John arrived armed with the instruction sheet and full of good intentions and seriously concerned for the health and welfare of John and Malcolm.

"The tower was going up fairly well."

"Should we check the strength of the wind?"

"Should the next bit be…?"

"The diagram says…"

"Are the fixings tight…?"

All this was met with nods, murmurs, OKs, given out at intervals as work continued slowly.

Mr Davis was now fully in site-foreman mode, gradually creeping nearer to the scaffold and desperately wanting to be a useful extra hand. However the 'labourers' were one step ahead of him and by now feeling quite efficient. Warnings were given for Mr D to be careful, not come too close to the tower, the boards being handed up weren't finally fixed into position etc. Would he listen? Oh no, he had the instructions. Next thing one board slips, John D goes one way and his spectacles go the other way. Once spectacles were retrieved and realigned he took the hint – the men could carry on without him and he found another project to get on with.

It is a testament to the friendship of the gang that when we sat down to another of Margaret's fine meals that night the job was near completion, John D was still in one piece and we were all still laughing. He was worried for a while though when Malcolm suggested he could paint the soffit and fascia if he stood on a chair on the tower! We all heard his sigh of relief when they admitted that that bit would need a professional painter.

The week continued with the odd visit to Tenby – the holiday break bit. This was usually armed with a shopping list for food, supplies and materials though. By now the holiday bit was long forgotten anyway as the McFalls were thoroughly enjoying themselves and it was like occupational therapy.

The week was turning out to be educational as well. At this time Laura was seriously into Ballamory and enjoyed watching several DVDs between her walks and kitchen supervising duties. A whole new experience for the Davis and McFall people. By the end of the week we certainly knew the tune and John McFall was starting to name the characters, much to Laura's amusement. Kit said, as we closed the gate on our way home, she was off to be deprogrammed. "What's the story Ballamory…" was a frequent tune in our heads that week.

There was one final treat in store – the Davis twosome invited the Melhuish and McFall families to an expedition into the Wheelabout's meadow. A picnic? No! Laura's wheelchair was fully charged, Malcolm and John McF were armed with spray paint cans and we were off to mark out a circular route for wheelchair access to the meadow. Laura was kitted out in a way that she could have taken on an arctic expedition – the sun was out but the heater wasn't working. She was thoroughly enjoying herself, laughing her head off. Perhaps it was something to do with the antics of the supposedly mature, responsible adults that she was surrounded by. Kit had the design of the meadow and the plan of the route in her head. The worker bees were instructed to peg out and mark the outline of the path which would be properly completed later on by someone else. Margaret and Laura were the ground-breaking adventurers trying out the route – a task that challenged every part of the wheelchair and Margaret's driving skills. More than once Malcolm had to help her out of a rut, or two, or three.

Our final night was a celebration of a wonderful week – Margaret, Laura and Kit excelled themselves in the kitchen. Jenny had been finally adopted by us whether she wanted to be or not, and was invited to join us. By now she was convinced that perhaps we were all certifiably mad though. Amid much hilarity we congratulated ourselves on our achievements. That was when John Davis calmly enquired if we'd enjoyed our break? Apparently it was a special activity holiday that not everyone gets.

So, beware, if John or Kit asks, quite innocently, if you'd like a day or two in Tenby – it could mean anything. It will mean though much fun, good companionship and another job or two well done!

CHAPTER 23

Finale

'Jumping o'er time
Turning the accomplishment of many years
Into an hour glass.'
William Shakespeare – *Henry V*

TWENTY YEARS IS quite a portion of our lives and not everything that has happened during that time has given us pleasure; like the fabled curate's egg it has been good in parts. Here then, in true competition style and in no particular order of preference or time, are some things we have enjoyed:

1   The excitement of the young boy on a visit to Giltar View to see if it would suit his disabled older brother. We went up to the attic bedrooms. He darted from one little single room (blue/ moon/ stars) "I'll have this one," to the other (yellow/ shells/ fishes). "No! I'll have this one." He looked at his mother and bounced excitedly, "I could bring a friend". Brothers and sisters often have to take a back seat and we have always tried to give support to the whole family.

2   Reading the cards and notes left for us.

3   Seeing the commitment of the staff at each house and in the office and the effort they make to ensure everything runs as smoothly as possible.

4   The chat and laughter we have shared with so many people.

5   Sharing a meal with trustees and friends.

6   The kindness of strangers and the help freely given to us, by people like Kevin Ayre who has guided us into the latest computer technology and who gives freely of his time and skills to organize the website.

7   Counting up 'the take' after a fund-raising event.

8   Seeing the mural in the swimming pool hall at the Wheelabout taking shape through the artistry of Jo and her friend Sandy, and being allowed to be an apprentice painter of seaweed. The lovely harbour scene in the lift shaft – designed, drawn and painted by Jo in her spare time.

9   A set of well-kept accounts – John.

10   Seeing the gardens and field at the Wheelabout and Caerwen flourish – Kit.

Amongst the less pleasant, more irritating or stressful things we count:

1   Sand in the washing machine or oil on a newly-laid carpet.

2   The boiler/central heating failing in the winter, especially late in the evening.

3   Calling the TV repairman/plumber yet again because the settings had been fiddled with.

4   Finding unreported damage or a dirty house at the end of a week (only rarely in 20 years and more than a thousand family holidays).

5   Being woken by a phone call early on Sunday morning and hearing the words: "Water's coming through the sitting room ceiling in Harriet's House, the Fire Brigade's here pumping it out."

6   Worrying about fund-raising/weeding/storm damage/ heating the pool.

7   Trying to prevent O_2 putting a Tetra mast yards from the Wheelabout garden – a failure, but what did we expect.

8   Not being able to fit in everyone who wants a holiday week or hearing that one of the special children has lost his or her struggle for life.

Harriet has been a hard taskmaster, but have we fulfilled her wish? What do the families who come to Harriet's House, Giltar View, the Wheelabout and Caerwen think? Are they like Shakespeare's Rosalind, "in a holiday humour"? Dip into the Visitors' Books and discover.

Harriet's House Visitors' Book Comments

Thank you so much for giving us the opportunity to enjoy a family holiday (the first one ever!) with J. (2004)

J has slept well all week (he usually has disturbed nights). (2005)

We have found our perfect holiday place. Many, many thanks. (2005)

What a week! Alice had measles, Harry a cold and Marley very poorly with a chest infection, but Harriet's is such a relaxing place who cared?! Asghar's first holiday and he really enjoyed the sea and soft play in the old church. We did manage a day to Folly Farm, what a fabulous bus service, great even for wheelchair users. Marley's first-ever bus ride. Hope to come to the wonderful home from home again. Thank you and best wishes to all that make this wonderful house available to special children and families every year. (2010)

Thank you for another wonderful holiday – in a house that is more suitable for our needs than our own! (2011)

J starts talking about his holiday to Tenby in January – home from home here – each year we go home more and more relaxed. Just what it should be (and what we all need). (2010)

We had a fantastic week, E was on great form and got plenty of fresh air – so easy looking after her in this house – makes such a difference x. (2011)

This is our first holiday M has had in 3 years since he had steel rods put in his back – thanks to the electric bed and he enjoyed the bath. (2004)

Giltar View Visitors' Book Comments

Good to see the house is as lovely and welcoming as it was when we last visited in 2002. (2011)

Fantastic house, home from home. Our twins have enjoyed themselves immensely and the adapted house has meant we have had a holiday ourselves. We are so grateful that this charity exists as what we always worried about planning a holiday has been overcome and hopefully we can continue to have such wonderful experiences. (2011)

S is very thankful that once again, due to the kindness of the H D Trust, he was able to bring the family for support, all the way from Lincolnshire, almost 300 miles away (with brother, Mum, Dad, aunt and uncle, Granny and Granddad). (2009)

We were so pleased to be back – the house was so welcoming with the Xmas decorations – thank you so much. (2008)

All enjoyed Tenby and the house. We found everything we needed and plenty of room. (2009)

Another lovely holiday (been coming for twelve years now, Yvonne – thanks for all your help). (2006)

Dear Kit, John, Yvonne and all at the Harriet Davis Trust: Thank you means you really didn't have to – but we are very grateful that you did. It also means that you have done something special that we will never ever forget. Thank you for allowing us to have our first family holiday in such a wonderful place. Our twins G and B are 10 today and have thoroughly enjoyed a stress-free holiday and so have we. Many thanks for this wonderful charity you have set up in memory of Harriet – a wonderful tribute x. (2011)

The Wheelabout Visitors' Book Comments

A great experience to know that there is somewhere we can take S and know there is special equipment for her and she coped so well with all her fears and phobias... Our elder daughter hasn't had a proper holiday before because of S's disabilities and she said she would not want to go anywhere other than back here. Not only for us but for Mum, Dad and brother, who has cerebral palsy. It has made us feel like a normal family. (2007)

This is the first hassle-free holiday and the first family holiday we have had for over ten years... D's beaming smile when being hoisted into the pool will stay with us forever. (2005)

S really appreciated all the disability aids in the bedroom – especially the tracked hoist and wow, what a bath! (2003)

Many thanks to Jo and Basil for a beautiful clean house x. (2007)

Friends of the M family – what a wonderful house and beautiful gardens – nice to spend time with W – and see him so happy. (2007)

Harriet Davis Trust! We all had a fantastic time. We take away with us memories of happy times and a longing to come back. (2011)

Harriet Davis Trust! We all had a fantastic holiday at the Wheelabout. Our six-year-old E had a fantastic time whizzing her wheelchair up and down the corridors and the lift was a firm favourite. E cannot stand or walk – she wanted you to know that whilst she was in the magic pool she learned to swim without armbands! It was such a big occasion! We explained to her that Mr & Mrs Davis set up the Trust and, as we left on Saturday, she looked at Harriet's photograph and said thank you! And so do we! (2011)

Caerwen Visitors' Book Comments

Just wanted to say thank you so much for allowing us to stay in this beautiful house. We have twin sons who are autistic and can be more than a handful. This house has enabled us to have a bit of a rest whilst our boys have jumped around the soft play area or worn themselves out running around the garden. We haven't had to watch them constantly because of the high fences and they have thoroughly enjoyed the freedom. The TV cabinet is fantastic and we have been able to relax knowing that our sons cannot constantly fiddle with the TV and DVD player. (2010)

We've all been so happy. This house is just great and has been safe, comfortable and a happy haven for a child like my son who has severe learning difficulties, autism and challenging behaviour. (2011)

A fabulous place to stay for a family with a severely autistic boy. Brilliantly designed and laid out. The soft play room was an eye opener. 'Tough' beds, home from home! Great to be able to lock the doors and actually sit down to a meal together for the first time on holiday for years without one of us on guard. (2011)

Thank you for such a wonderful holiday. The house is so clean, safe and most of all relaxing. We finally had a couple of nights' sleep. E loved the playroom. (2007)

We had a wonderful holiday here at this lovely house. The boys settled in immediately, a first for them, a big part to play in that is the playroom – it's a brilliant innovative idea. As parents we have been able to relax knowing that the boys are in a secure and safe environment. (2007)

Thank you for the most relaxing holiday we have ever had. The house is so inviting, safe and secure. As 'Mum' holidays are usually just a change of walls with extra guard duties, but this year I have had a break and a sleep! (2007)

We have enjoyed a marvellous week. The house is spacious, comfortable and thoughtfully fitted out and has helped us to relax. R, aged 7, soon felt at home and very secure. (2007)

The playroom was a masterstroke, the children have played calmly all week. (2008)

I would recommend this house to anyone I know with children with additional needs. (2008)

The fact that it is away from neighbours meant that Ben could make lots of noise. (2008)

The house made all the difference to the children, they settled in immediately and it was good to have such a good base to explore Pembrokeshire. From our point of view it was nice to be able to relax in a house that was tailored to their needs knowing that they were safe to enjoy themselves. (2008)

We were given details of Caerwen by a close friend who works at a special educational needs school. We booked Caerwen, virtually on return home. We had never holidayed away from home previously... it was indeed a wondrous experience. (2009)

When Harriet died we found it difficult to make sense of all that had happened to us after her birth in 1980, and we struggled to reshape our philosophy of life in order to look to a future so different from what, in 1979, we had imagined it would be. Reading the comments written by families who have used the Trust houses, is perhaps all we should need as answers to our questioning.

Kit and John Davis
Begelly
June 2012

APPENDIX

Trees and wild flowers in the Star Meadow

Trees in the Hedgerows

Common Ash	*Fraxinus excelsior*
Common Hawthorn	*Crataegus monogyna*
Blackthorn	*Frangula alnus*
Buckthorn Alder	*Alder alnus*

New Planting

Purple-leaved Sycamore	*Acer psuedoplatanus purpureum*
Eastern Thorn	*Crataegus laciniata*
Common Whitebeam	*Sorbus aria*
Silver-leaved Whitebeam	*Sorbus aria lutescens*
Mountain Ash	*Sorbus aucuparia*
Midland Hawthorn	*Crataegus laevigata*
Hawthorn Paul's Scarlet	*Spicrataegus laevigata*
Common Hawthorn	*Crataegus monogyna*
Rowan Chinese Lace	*Sorbus hupehensis*
Wild Service Tree	*Sorbus torminalis*
Bird Cherry	*Prunuspadus*
Wild Cherry or Gean	*Prunus avium*
Damson Shropshire Prune	*Prunus damascena*
Majestic Whitebeam	*Sorbus aria majestic*
Field Maple	*Acer campestres*
Hornbeam	*Carpinus betulus*
Weeping Ash	*Fraxinus excelsior pendula*

Crab Apple Tree Golden Hornet *Malus sylvestris*
Apple Devon Queenie *Malus*
Apple Peter's Pippin *Malus*

Conifers
Common Spruce *Picea abies*
Austrian Pine *Pinus nigra*
Monteray Pine *Pinus radiata*

Some of the wildflowers
Bluebell, bramble, common daisy, cuckoo pint, curled dock, dog rose, ferns in variety, field scabious, foxgloves, goose grass, greater knapweed, hemp agrimony, honeysuckle, ivy, lesser celadine, meadow buttercup, meadowsweet, nettle, oxeye daisy, primroses, purple vetch, ragwort, red clover, rib wort, rosebay willow-herb, speedwell, tufted vetch, white clover, wild celery, wild hop, wild parsley, yellow vetch.

Grasses
Creeping bent, rye grass, sheep's fescue, timothy, Yorkshire fog.

PLAN OF THE WHEELABOUT AND STAR MEADOW

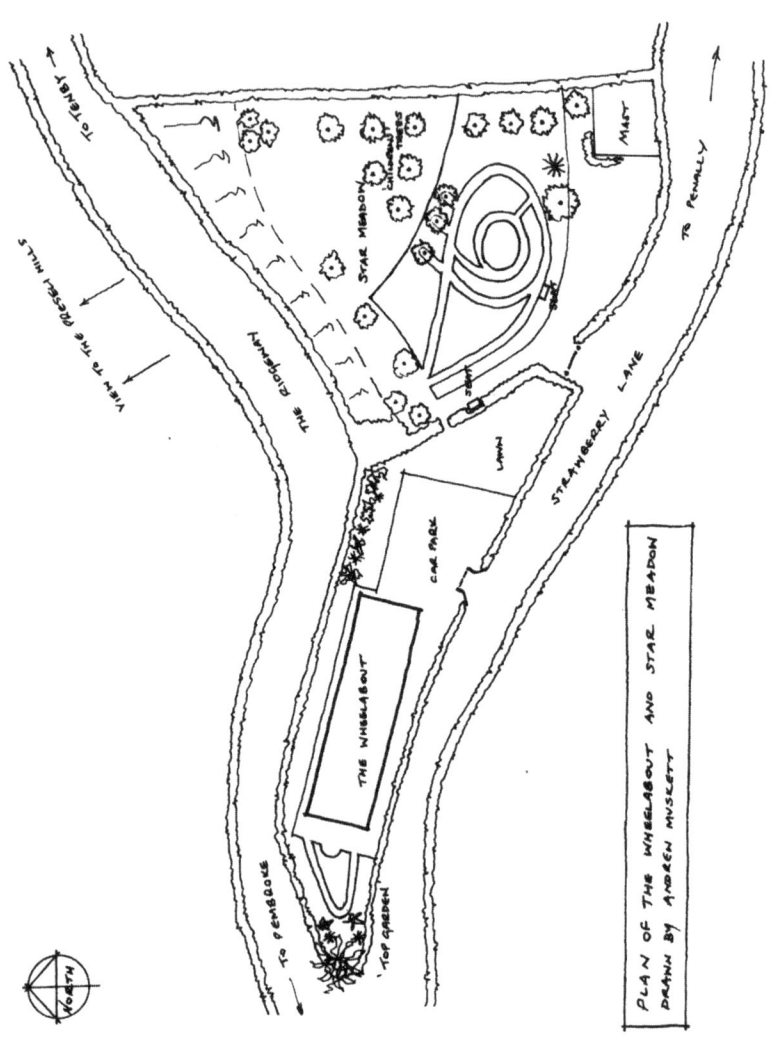

TO FOREST

VIEW TO THE PRESELI HILLS

STAR MEADOW

THE GLOUCESTER?

MARY

TO PENALLY

STRAWBERRY LANE

LAWN

CAR PARK

THE WHEELABOUT

TO PEMBROKE

TOP GARDEN

NORTH

PLAN OF THE WHEELABOUT AND STAR MEADOW
DRAWN BY ANDREW MUSKETT

ACKNOWLEDGEMENTS

Blissymbols reproduced by kind permission of Blissymbolics Communication International (www.blissymbolics.org).

Programme notes from the play *Glory! Glory! Diolch Iddo* quoted by kind permission of Tony Jasper.

BIBLIOGRAPHY

Dewi Davies, *Welsh Place Names and their Meanings* (2011).

Gwili Gog, *Understanding Welsh Place Names* (2010).

Duchess of Hamilton and Christopher Humphreys, *Native Trees and Shrubs for your Garden* (2005).

From Harriet with Love is just one of a whole range of publications from Y Lolfa. For a full list of books currently in print, send now for your free copy of our new full-colour catalogue. Or simply surf into our website

www.ylolfa.com

for secure on-line ordering.

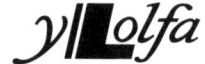

TALYBONT CEREDIGION CYMRU SY24 5HE
e-mail ylolfa@ylolfa.com
website www.ylolfa.com
phone (01970) 832 304
fax 832 782